The Practice of Concern

Carolina Academic Press
Ethnographic Studies in Medical Anthropolgy Series

Pamela J. Stewart
and
Andrew Strathern
Series Editors

The Practice of Concern

Ritual, Well-Being, and Aging in Rural Japan

John W. Traphagan

Department of Asian Studies and Population Research Center
University of Texas at Austin

CAROLINA ACADEMIC PRESS
Durham, North Carolina

Library of Congress Cataloging-in-Publication Data

Traphagan, John W.
The practice of concern : ritual, well-being, and againg in rural
Japan / by John W. Traphagan.
    p.   cm.
Includes bibliographical references.
ISBN 0-89089-406-X
    1. Aged—Japan. 2. Aging—Japan. 3. Aged—Religious life—Japan.
4. Aged—Health and hygeine—Japan. 5. Aged—Japan—Social life and
customs. 6. Rites and ceremonies—Japan. I. Title.

HQ1064.J3T72 2003
305.26'0952—dc22   2003065291

CAROLINA ACADEMIC PRESS
700 Kent Street
Durham, North Carolina 27701
Telephone (919) 489-7486
Fax (919) 493-5668
www.cap-press.com

Printed in the United States of America

For Mom, who will be greatly missed

Contents

Medical Anthropology Series Editors' Preface

Pamela J. Stewart and Andrew Strathern

This is an extremely well-rounded, mature, and professionally written book, solidly based on extensive fieldwork and careful analysis of the relevant Japanese behavioral responses regarding aging processes. The author's overall approach is encapsulated neatly in the title: *The Practice of Concern: Ritual, Well-Being, and Aging in Rural Japan*. Old age and its associated transformations in health, general well-being, and family relationships, is an object of concern among people everywhere and has been throughout time. The Greek mythological tale of Tithonus (a mortal who fell in love with the goddess Dawn) dramatically depicts the fate of prolonged life and aging. In this classic story Tithonus, the son of a king of Troy, was granted the gift of living forever but he was not also provided with eternal youth. Thus, as time passed Tithonus grew older, weaker, and less mobile but did not pass onward to the next phase of the cycle of existence, i.e., death.

Many of the discussions in *The Practice of Concern* are ones that are also applicable to contexts outside of Japan, e.g., the U.S.A. Debates over health care, availability of medical supplies, and quality of life for "Seniors" are major political and social concerns. Traphagan's detailed study explores the way people in his study area deal with these concerns through particular ritual practices that both the aging and their kin or community members undertake in order to cope with the particular circumstances of aging itself. The effect of this approach is that the author's text illuminates both Japanese ideas of religion, seen through the lens of ritual practices, and the specific concepts regarding aging and well being, such as "ikigai" (self-discipline) counterposed against "boke" (loss of self). Dealing with aging, and keeping well-being always in sight, leads to "omairi", the practice of concern.

One of the excellent features of this book is its general blending of different modes of analysis. Cultural meanings are explicated along with sociological and ethnographic descriptions of data, and the works of Japanese specialists are juxtaposed with those of theorists such as Paul Connerton on memory and Michel Foucault on discourse. This strategy of writing leads to an account that is well adapted to use both by researchers working in the field of gerontology and by students, graduate or undergraduate, seeking to gain a grasp of Japanese culture and society and in general to understand the intersection of religion and ritual in healing practices.

Traphagan's perspectives on themes in Japanese society show this same ability to project a balanced narrative. An example is his handling of the distinction between Shinto and Buddhism, where he writes that "the post-Meiji Restoration separation of institutional Shinto and Buddhism was something imposed by political authorities rather than inherent in the ways people historically have practiced the two religions." Or on kinship relations, where he considers the persistence of the stem-family as a family ideal and points out that nowadays this only "intensifies the distancing older people feel in rural areas," because of the shift from a three-generational to a two-generational nuclear family structure. Traphagan is also able to illuminate relations of a personal kind with ancestors, pointing out how "feelings of close relationships between the living and the dead appear to become stronger when one has experienced the death of a close relative." He also notes that for the elderly, "the tutelary power of the ancestors over their descendants continues to be important," while this is less the case for younger people. Very interesting here is Traphagan's treatment of dreams, and how these enter into people's ideas of relations with ancestors and one another. If someone has an accident in the family, ancestors may appear in dreams to their kins-folk as a sign of their care for their descendants. Similar ideas about kin appearing in dreams occur in many other societies (see Lohmann 2003 for a recent collection of essays on this topic).

As a contribution to the literature on both gerontology in partic-ular and medical anthropology in general, this book is distinguished by its holistic approach. The author places old age into the overall practices of ritual and the exercise of concern for well-being. Fol-lowing the insights of Emiko Ohnuki-Tierney and Margaret Lock he also sets the issue of illness into the cosmic notions of balance, in which the aim of therapy is not to attain perfect health but to restore a balance that has been disturbed. He points out that women have a particular obligation as caretakers for the elderly. This raises the in-teresting question of what role is accorded to such women as ances-tors when they themselves die. Senior women as care-givers occupy a kind of "healer" role. This is not unlike examples from other soci-eties where women find themselves responsible for care-giving to eld-erly family members while also balancing their lives in terms of work, children and spouses. Not all processes have a harmonious outcome. Traphagan points out that as a result of demographic and economic changes in some areas older people may live in solitude and younger people may resent the role of taking care for the aged. The incidence of suicide points to strains of this sort in familial relations. In gen-eral, however, women themselves take on special care-giving roles in the family structure, and Traphagan strikingly suggests that they be-come like priestesses of the inner domestic world while men play major roles in "matsuri," public collective rituals. Such an analysis projects the idea of the complementarity of ritual functions as basic to gender relations (see Stewart and Strathern 1999, 2002 for exam-ples of this process of complementarity in Papua New Guinean con-texts).

Another strength of Traphagan's book is its dual focus on personal, intimate rituals and public expressions of collective concern. The au-thor analyzes the roles of elders in collective rituals as personifications of concern for the community. By their ritual actions they purify themselves and thus also strengthen the community as a whole. Thus, the rituals performed purify the whole community. This analysis has the intriguing outcome of suggesting that the whole schema of purity and pollution is a means of articulating concern for the community, not just in terms of its boundaries but as a means of ensuring its well-being. Individuals may also harness the purifying power for their own therapeutic purposes. While avoiding any stereotypical "groupist" characterization of Japanese social relations, Traphagan succeeds in showing how "the boundaries between individual, family, and community are not necessarily sharply drawn in the Japanese way of looking at the world."

This fine study is a significant contribution to gerontology, Japanese studies, religious studies, and medical anthropology, and it is a delight to read in terms of its careful modes of presentation and vigorous narrative as well as theoretical and analytical conclusions. The book clearly addresses the role of religion and ritual in healing practices and could profitably be used as a textbook in courses on religious studies, medical anthropology, and introductory cultural anthropology.

We are very pleased to present John Traphagan's book as the most recent contribution to the Ethnographic Studies in Medical Anthropology Series. The other titles in this Series include:

"*Curing and Healing: Medical Anthropology in Global Perspective*", 1999 (by Andrew Strathern and Pamela J. Stewart)

"*Healing the Modern in a Central Javanese City*", 2001 (by Steve Ferzacca)

"*Physicians at Work, Patients in Pain: Biomedical Practice and Patient Response in Mexico*, 2nd edition" 2001 (by Kaja Finkler)

"*Elusive Fragments: Making Power, Propriety, and Health in Samoa*", 2002 (by Douglass Drozdow-St. Christian)

"*Endangered Species: Health, Illness, and Death among Madagascar's People of the Forest*" 2002 (by Janice Harper)

References

Lohmann, Roger, ed. (2003) *Dream Travelers: Sleep Experiences and Culture in the Western Pacific.* New York and London: Palgrave Macmillan.

Stewart, Pamela J. and Andrew Strathern (1999) Female Spirit Cults as a Window on Gender Relations in the Highlands of Papua New Guinea. *The Journal of the Royal Anthropological Institute* 5(3):345–360.

Stewart, Pamela J. and A. Strathern (2002) *Gender, Song, and Sensibility: Folktales and Folksongs in the Highlands of New Guinea.* Westport, CT and London: Praeger (Greenwood Publishing).

September 2003
Department of Anthropology
University of Pittsburgh
Pittsburgh, PA 15260 USA

Acknowledgments

Many people have been helpful in the fieldwork that went into this book and in commenting on the thinking that accompanied its writing. I wish to first thank Andrew Strathern and Pamela Stewart who kindly asked if I had any interesting data that might fit into this series on medical anthropology. I have been very fortunate to have the opportunity to know Dr. Strathern and to learn a great deal about anthropology from him over the years, and it is difficult to adequately put into words how much I appreciate his encouragement and support. I would also like to thank L. Keith Brown, Christopher Ellison, Akiko Hashimoto, Tamotsu Kawamura, Susan O. Long, Hikaru Suzuki, Jeanne Traphagan, Tomoko Traphagan, Willis Traphagan, and Jan Zeserson, who read and commented upon various drafts of the manuscript or helped with other aspects of the writing. And many thanks go to John Mock for his generous help in arranging housing and providing contacts for the Akita portion of the research. I am also very appreciative of my colleagues in the Department of Asian Studies and the Population Research Center at the University of Texas at Austin, who have provided many hours of intellectual discourse that have influenced the contents of this volume. Most of all, I want to thank the people of Kanegasaki, Mizusawa, and Akita who have given a great deal of their time to me so that I can learn about their lives.

Funding for fieldwork and writing for this book was provided by a variety of sources. Fieldwork in 1995 and 1996 was supported by a Fulbright Doctoral Research Grant and in 1998 by grants from the Northeast Asia Council of the Association for Asian Studies, the Michigan Exploratory Center for the Demography of Aging, and the

Wenner-Gren Foundation for Anthropological Research. A major portion of the research for this book was supported by grant AG016111 on Religion, Well-Being, and Aging in Japan, from the National Institute on Aging and follow-up trips were supported by the Mitsubishi Endowment Fund in the Department of Asian Studies at the University of Texas at Austin. Finally, writing was supported by a Summer Research Assistance grant from the University of Texas at Austin. I am very grateful to all of these organizations for their support of my work. Portions of chapters 2, 4, 5, and 6 appeared in earlier forms in the *Journal of Anthropological Research* (2000b), *Ethnology* (2003b), and the *Journal of Cross-Cultural Gerontology* (2000c) and are included here with permission of these journals.

A Note on Conventions

All names of Japanese individuals in this book are presented using the Japanese custom of writing the family name before the given name. As is common in ethnographic writing, the names of all individuals who participated in the research have been changed to protect their identities. In some cases, interview data from specific individuals appear in more than one of my published works; in these instances, names of individuals across publications are sometimes intentionally inconsistent in order to provide as much protection of the individual's identity as possible. Romanization throughout the book follows the Hepburn system.

Map of Japan

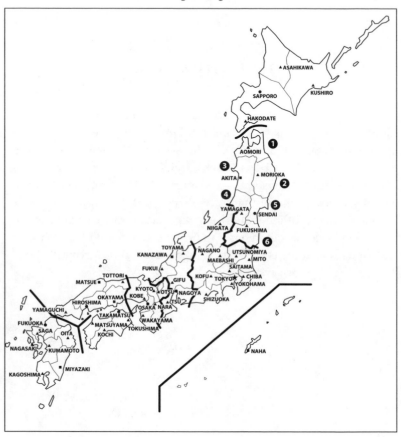

The Tōhoku region of Japan consists of Aomori (1), Iwate (2), Akita (3), Yamagata (4), Miyagi (5), and Fukushima (6) Prefectures.

The Practice of Concern

Chapter 1

Introduction

New Year's Day, 1996

If you visit a shrine on New Year's morning for
three consecutive years, you won't get sick.

—(in Brown 1979:218)

*New Year's eve capped a busy day at the farm. The morning had been
spent cleaning the house* (susuharai) *to remove the previous year's dirt
and to purify the home for the coming year. Women stood in the kitchen
throughout the day, sending the warming smells of traditional New
Year's dishes throughout the house. Ozōni, a soup in which* omochi *(rice
cakes) are placed along with burdock roots* (gobō), *cooked on the stove.
Mandarin oranges* (mikan), *rice crackers, cakes, and many other foods
appeared throughout the day on the kitchen table as snacks for the family members who sat, smoked, and talked. The evening's supper had consisted of buckwheat noodles* (soba), *symbolizing long life and the hope
that all in the family would be well in the coming year. At midnight we
could hear in the distance the bell from a local temple toll 108 times (representing the 108 human sins identified in Buddhism). Later we visited
the neighborhood Shintō shrine in order to ring in the New Year with
our requests for a good year and to make offerings of a few coins to the
deity. On the morning of New Year's day, I skipped the reading of New
Year's cards* (nengajō) *that people enjoy as soon as the postman arrives
and drove across town to attend a ceremony at Kanegasaki Jinja, a
Shintō shrine located in the park along the Kitakami River. Along with*

the New Year, the previous night had brought several centimeters of fresh snow accompanied by a strong wind that blew the snow across the streets causing occasional white-outs and making driving even more hazardous than usual on the ice-covered roads.

After about thirty minutes, I turned down the one-lane street—a gravel road with concrete walls on either side, making it impossible for more than one car to pass at a time—parked the car, and headed to the shrine on foot. Moving carefully across the ice and snow covered roads, I soon approached the shrine, an old, wooden building with a faded red roof that is set amongst cherry trees on a knoll overlooking the river. The gray, leafless trees blended into the old, weathered wood of the building and the entire frigid scene merged into the overcast tones of the wintry sky. The wind was blowing hard and heavy snow started to fall as people, bundled up to keep out the cold wind, rushed to get inside.

As groups and individuals arrived at the shrine, they stopped before the rope and bell that hang at the entrance, as is normal at most Shintō shrines, to briefly pray before the deity. There was little uniformity to the manner in which people engaged in this customary behavior. Some rang the bell first, bowed, and then clapped. Some bowed twice, some only once. Some didn't ring the bell at all, perhaps wanting to escape the cold and enter the shrine building as quickly as possible.

Following this brief homage to the deity of the shrine, the participants removed their boots and overcoats and entered the building. All in attendance were wearing their "Sunday best." The men were dressed in gray, blue, or blue pinstripe suits and virtually all were wearing ties. There were perhaps three or four women (all over the age of sixty-five) in attendance as regular participants; the other three women were working. Two of the working women were shrine maidens (miko) dressed in white robes, and the other was a woman who works for the local community center who was helping to move some of the furniture and other objects in the room. The other participants, about forty altogether, were men.

Everyone sat on the tatami *mats that covered the floor, in the middle of which had been placed two large kerosene heaters to fight off the winter chill in this otherwise unheated building. The ceremony included people from the area of town known as the Machichiku district, which consists of three neighborhoods in the center of Kanegasaki—Honchō,*

Suwa-kōji, and Jōnai. As I looked around the room it was readily evident that apart from myself, the only other younger men were the assistant director of the community center and the head of the fire brigade, who came wearing part of his fireman's uniform—a happi *coat-over his shirt and tie. Other than these two men, myself, and the mayor, who lives in the Honchō neighborhood, and who was in his mid-fifties at the time, there were no other men under the age of sixty-five in attendance. Most appeared to be in their seventies, a fact that was confirmed as I looked at several of the men I knew—Itoh Hiroshi (73), Fukuwara Owari (78), Fujii Seiko (77), and Inoue Tadashi (70), who was the head of the Self-Government Association* (jichikai) *for Jōnai, the neighborhood in which I lived.*

As we awaited the beginning of the ceremony, we huddled around the kerosene stoves for warmth. The air became increasingly unpleasant as the stoves produced a parched heat accompanied by the odor of burning kerosene. The discomfort of the air was intensified by the fact that several of the men lit cigarettes, adding a thick haze of smoke and the pungent aroma of strong tobacco to the acrid smell of the kerosene. The men sat separately from the women, who were in another part of the room, somewhat remote from the heaters. Everyone was chatting—mostly about the snow and cold wind, which was rattling the sliding doors of the building and blowing into the room. At one point, a strong gust of wind suddenly blasted through the building, causing everyone to shudder. More participants entered, and some dropped to their knees to bow with their hands in front of them and their heads to the floor saying "akemashite omedetō gozaimasu," the Japanese equivalent of Happy New Year, to those already in the room. Others simply came in, sat down, and started smoking.

The main room of the shrine looked as though it had been recently refurbished. Some of the paneling on the walls appeared to be new and the floor of the altar appeared newly refinished. At the center of the room, on the wall near the ceiling over the entrance to the area in which the altar was placed, a sign had been hung that said Kanegasaki Jinja, written horizontally from right to left. Bottles of saké were placed to the right of the altar in the central sacred area of the room; after the ceremony, and after the bottles had been purified by the priest, these were given to the important men in attendance, all prominent figures in town politics.

After about twenty minutes, the director of the community center—Matsumoto Junichi—got up and began to request our attention. The din subsided, cigarettes were extinguished, and everyone moved to a formal position sitting on their legs, with back upright and hands resting on the tops of their thighs (seiza). Matsumoto was a man of 69 years who had worked in the town government most of his life and, upon mandatory retirement, had been given a part-time post as the director of the community center in Honchō. As such, he was among the most important men in the community, continuing to hold a government post after retirement, and always one of the main figures in any kind of local meeting. On this day, his role was that of master of ceremonies, managing the flow of short speeches (aisatsu) that usually begins formal and many informal public gatherings in Japan. Matsumoto commenced the ceremony by wishing everyone Happy New Year and complimenting them on the success of another year gone by. After a few words of encouragement for the New Year, the head of the town's Board of Education rose to offer a few more words of encouragement for the year to come. Short speeches continued as various prominent men, such as the directors of the Self-Government Associations from each neighborhood, offered a few words. Finally, after what seemed like a very long time, the head of the rengōkai (the Unity Association which includes the heads of each of the Self-Government Associations in the district) gave the last speech, juxtaposing life in Kanegasaki against the tumultuous national events of the previous year:

> It has been a difficult year for Japan and it seems as though there is a dark atmosphere hanging over the country. We experienced the gassing of the subway in Tokyo by Aum as well as the great earthquake in Kobe. But things have been very positive in Kanegasaki. The opening of the new Town Hall and the big celebration for the 40th anniversary of the town's amalgamation [from several villages into a larger municipality] are a few examples.

After the speeches, the priest, dressed in his robes of white and light blue, who had been sitting in the seiza position to the left and front of the central sacred area waiting for his turn in the ceremony as the old

*men spoke, slowly and deliberately began the chanting and prayer that
was at the center of the ceremony. He struck a large wooden drum with
the head placed vertically to his right in a rhythm that started slowly
and became increasingly fast and loud, ending in a decrescendo as he
reached the highest tempo. The drum, according to the priest of this
shrine, is used to alert the people in attendance that the ceremony has
begun, but it also is used as a means of calming the* kokoro *or cen-
ter/mind of those participating, allowing them to focus their attention
on the ceremony. Following the drum, he began chanting a request to the
deities for protection in the coming year, at which point all in attendance
bowed deeply while kneeling and resting palms down flat on the floor in
front of them. After the chanting, the priest took a stack of* sakaki
*branches with white paper streamers attached to them and gave one to
each of the headmen, who were all sitting on an electrically heated carpet at the center and front of the room, just before the sacred area.*

*As each man received a branch, he stood and took it to the altar,
turned it in the opposite direction from which he had been given it, and
placed it on the altar. The first man to do this was the head of the*
rengōkai, *followed by the mayor, and then the other men on the carpet.
As they returned to the heated carpet, each of the men bowed once to the
priest and then once to the rest of us in the room.*

After the last man sat down, the priest took the oharai (*or* nusa,
which is the technical term in Shintō, although most priests use oharai),
*a long stick with paper streamers attached to one end, and waved it over
the deity, which was placed in the back of the sacred space. Following
this, he waved it over the saké and then over the people in attendance,
focusing on the men on the heated carpet, as all in attendance bowed.*[1]
The priest then returned the oharai *to its stand and knelt to begin a second round of chanting, during which all in attendance again bowed
deeply. Finally, the priest moved to the drum and started the same ca-
dence of slow to fast, bringing his portion of the ceremony to a close with
the final decrescendo of the drum.*

*The head of the Board of Education stood up and announced that the
ceremony was complete, following which people started to open bottles
of sake and bring out boxes of* mikan. *Within only a few minutes, many
of the men were beginning to behave in a moderately drunken way, talk-*

ing loudly, smoking, and laughing a great deal. They drank saké that had been made in Iwate Prefecture, where Kanegasaki is located; the saké that had been opened and poured was from the stock that was purified by the priest during the course of the ceremony, providing an opportunity for participants to literally embody the renewal and purification associated with the ritual.

What was clear, as the ceremony progressed, was that in many ways the ritual performance was focused upon the men sitting on the heated carpet; although all in attendance were being purified through the actions of the priest, it was obvious that these men were particularly important as community leaders and, thus, were the focus of the purification ceremony. Their participation as representatives of the community, as well as the participation of others as representatives of their households, extended the purification beyond the confines of the room to the community as a whole. This brief ceremony, in which elder men took center stage, was an important event in maintaining the well-being not only of the individuals in attendance, but of the collectivity of which they were a part and which they represented.

The men continued to drink for about fifteen or twenty minutes, after which they started to leave the shrine, gathering their coats and heading back into the cold wind and snow. While I walked back to my car, I passed other people who were coming to the shrine to ring the bell and throw some money or rice into the box in front of the shrine as an offering to the deity. Most of these people were younger than those who had participated in the morning ritual and many of them were women or young families.

I had been living in Kanegasaki for about a year when this New Year's ceremony took place. I arrived in the village of Jōnai just after New Year's in 1995 to conduct ethnographic fieldwork about the activities of older people in Japan. My initial aim had been to look at how people use facilities such as community centers to keep active as they make the transition from middle age to old age. However, as I continued my fieldwork, I came to understand that community centers and the activities pursued within them formed a web of symbols through which people engaged and interpreted meanings related to the aging process and to moral behavior. When asked, older people invariably responded that they involved themselves in activities at the community center or elsewhere—activities such as tea ceremony, gateball (a game similar to croquet), or *go*—to avoid the onset of senility (*boke*). At a most basic level, the hobbies and other activities in which older people involved themselves were forms of preemptive medicine designed and intended to help with the prevention of cognitive and physical decline. They also formed a pedagogy of agency used to aid in the retention of a cultural memory connected with the morality of action that identifies what it means to be human in Japan—the loss or forgetting of this cultural memory being closely associated with the experience and interpretation of senility.

After returning to the United States, and reflecting on and analyzing the fieldnotes and other forms of data I had collected in Japan, it became increasingly clear that many activities of older people were directed toward the aim of maintaining well-being. This well-being was conceptualized not only in the form of individual physical and mental health, but also the collective well-being of the families and communities in which my informants lived, and through these activities hopefully avoided or delayed the onset of senility. Building upon Lawrence Cohen's (1998) theoretical work dealing with the cultural construction of senility in India, in particular, I argued that senility was not simply a biomedical category in Japan, but a moral concept closely related to Japanese ideas about the good person defined in terms of activity (Traphagan 2000a). To be a good person—and particularly to be a good *rōjin* (old person)—is to be a socially engaged individual who is involved in activities that incorporate social interaction; failure to maintain activity and social involvement invites loss of well-being and, for the elderly, the onset of senility.

I will use the term '*rōjin*' throughout this book, but it is important to recognize that there are several terms frequently used in Japanese to identify the elderly. Terms such as *kōreisha, toshiyori,* or *nenpai* are a few of the possibilities, and it is common for Japanese to refer to elderly people as either Grandma or Grandpa (*obā-san* or *ojī-san*) even when there is no relation. My focus on the term *rōjin* is based upon two points. First, this is the term typically used by the government to identify the elderly, or those who are over the age of 65. The term, however, is not neutral—many elderly see the term as having a negative connotation because it directly references agedness (See Traphagan 1998c, 2000a). Although there is a growing tendency to use *kōreisha*, which is presented as having a less negative connotation, *rōjin* is still very widely used, particularly when referring to institutional contexts such as the *rōjin kurabu* (Old Persons Club discussed in chapter 6) or nursing homes (*rōjin hōmu*). Second, because of its negative connotation, the term implies a sense of social differentiation of the elderly as a class of people. This is particularly important in the Japanese context, because such differentiation is at once seen as legitimate by many in society while often, but by no means always, being contested by the elderly themselves.

The central point in *Taming Oblivion* was that there is a moral component of functional decline in old age, because there is a sense that individuals have some degree of control over that decline, even while there is a clear awareness that an individual may not be able to maintain that control as a condition, such as Alzheimer's disease, develops. The moral element lies in the idea that one should continually be making every effort possible to prevent the onset of functional decline; if that decline begins, there is at least the suggestion that one may not have made sufficient efforts to prevent or delay it. The activities older people use in their efforts to delay function decline— most of which Americans would place in the category of hobbies— are one way in which they attempt to manage the social and physical processes associated with the aging body. As I considered my field-notes, and thought more about aging in Japan through a second trip for fieldwork in 1998, I came to the conclusion that another context in which people engage in actions aimed at maintaining health and well-being is that associated with religiously oriented ritual and ceremonial practice.[2]

As I looked into the topic of religion and aging, I found that, while there was a growing literature within the social sciences on the topic, most of the research had been done in the U.S. and virtually none of it had been ethnographic in nature. Culture had not found its way deeply into the literature. Questions such as, "Do people pray more when they get old?" had been asked, but questions such as, "Do people conceptualize prayer differently as they age and how does culture influence the meaning of prayer?" or "How are religion or well-being cultural constructs?" had not been asked. In the ethnographic vignette that opens this chapter, we can see that one way in which religion and aging are closely tied together in Japan is through age hierarchies. It is the old who are often charged with the responsibility of attending and conducting ritual and ceremonial performances at temples and shrines. At New Year's, for example, it is old men, and a few old women, who attend the ceremony and accept the purification of the priest as representatives of their respective households and the community more broadly.[3] It is not considered necessary for everyone in the household to attend the ceremony or visit the shrine. Nor is it necessary that the representative be the eldest male in the household. But far more often than not, it is the eldest male in a household who attends such services, followed by the eldest female if there is no capable or living male, and it is this representative who receives the purification conveyed by the priest to him and by extension to the household and community he represents. The elderly are not only the ones primarily charged with the work of ritual performance, they are also the ones charged with maintaining the collective well-being, through ritual, of their families and of the communities in which they live. This is accomplished through a combination of private and public "prayer" activities that are central aspects of Japanese religious life.

What I hope to make clear throughout this book is that it is this ritual and ceremonial activity itself that matters most for Japanese, rather than a set of specific beliefs related to gods, spirits, or other entities. This recognition has important implications for research into the intersection of religion, health, and aging, because it indicates the need for a shift away from the conceptualizations of religion—largely centering on concepts of belief, faith, forgiveness, etc.—that have shaped much of the work in this area to date. I will return to this point in the next chapter as I discuss the manner in which "religion" has been approached in the gerontological literature and the inability of this approach to address issues of religion and aging in Japan.

Culture, Religion, and Aging

The perspectives I will develop in this volume center around a specific assumption: that an investigation into the role of religion or spirituality in the aging process necessitates situating that process within cultural context.[4] By culture, I mean learned behaviors and ideas that humans acquire, create, and contest as members of a society, and which they *interpret* as in some way defining the characteristics and parameters of that society and unifying the people who live within it. I emphasize interpret here because the fact that people often interpret their own and other cultures as bounded things should not be transferred to the use of culture as an analytic concept. Because at its root culture is a product of interpretation and invention, from an analytic perspective it cannot be understood in terms of tidy boundaries, nor can it be reified to neatly represent the behaviors or ideas of a particular society, even while many or most within that society may, in fact, represent themselves in a very unified way.

As Rappaport (1999:9) writes, every "human society develops a unique culture, which is also to say that it constructs a unique world that includes...a special understanding" of the world its members inhabit. In other words, all humans, by virtue of membership in a society, inhabit a cultural frame that shapes the way in which they look at the world. Ideas related to religion, health, well-being, and aging are generated within these frames, and thus should not be seen as jibing or running parallel across different societies. Recognizing the importance of culture in relation to the study of religion, health, and aging—particularly if we want to understand the intersection of these concepts[5] across cultural, ethnic, and sectarian boundaries—has important consequences for research, because it forces us to recognize the need to question our own assumptions about the nature of religious or spiritual behavior, health and illness, or what constitutes religion itself. The study of Japanese religious and ritual behavior is particularly appropriate for challenging preconceptions about the relationship between religion, health, and aging precisely because Japanese, in general, do not organize their religious behaviors around notions of faith or belief as is common in North American religious groups. While religious behavior, particularly religious ritual behavior, is evident and significant in both Western and Japanese societies, the assumptions upon which religious behavior is based—ideas about its function and form—are very different.

When it comes to the elderly, one aspect that Japanese and American religions appear to share is higher levels of participation in ritual and other activities among older populations. Survey research on the religiosity of Americans has indicated that older Americans generally rate religion as a very important part of their lives. As Susan McFadden points out, national surveys conducted by the Princeton Religion Research Center indicate that approximately 76 percent of older Americans view religion as very important in their lives, 52 percent of those over 65 regularly attend religious services, and 64 percent watch religious programs on the television (McFadden 1995:162). By comparison, a 1981 survey on "The Religious Consciousness of the Japanese", conducted by NHK Broadcasting Corporation, showed that there may be a strong age effect on beliefs in both Shintō and Buddhist deities. Only 28 percent (for Shinto *kami*) and 31 percent (for Buddhist *hotoke*) of people at age 20 indicated that they either were certain or accepted the possibility that these deities existed. But there is a steady increase in this affirmation until it reaches 65 percent and 48 percent, respectively, by age 70 (Swyngedouw 1993:52).

The difficulty in making sense out of a comparison of religious behavior among older (or other) Japanese and Americans, and, by extension drawing conclusions that apply across different cultural contexts, lies in addressing the question: What is meant by religion? In most of the literature on religions and aging, religion is equated with Judaism and Christianity. Research on religious behavior in old age has looked at topics such as indicators of religiosity as predictors of life satisfaction in later life (Markides, Levin, and Ray 1987) or the relationship between religious activity and physical functioning among the elderly (Haley, Koenig and Bruchett 2001), but has given only limited attention to the nature of the thing they are studying—particularly as it is culturally constructed in various contexts (see Musick et al. 2000).

Within gerontological writing, two terms have been widely used to refer to a set of practices and beliefs that typically fall into the scope of "religiosity"—spirituality and religion. Some researchers have noted that it is necessary to distinguish between what is meant by "spirituality" and "religion", recognizing that people may identify themselves as spiritual while eschewing participation in religion or religious institutions. Some authors advocate a universal "definition of spirituality that encompasses religious and nonreligious perspectives" (Anandarajah and Hight 2001:82), largely ignoring the fact that in some societies, such as Japan, people may routinely engage religious institutions without expressing much concern over the spiritual content related to the activities—the rituals, festivals, and ceremonies—they perform. A brief list of the variety of terms used in the attempt to represent these forms of behavior in the gerontological corpus on religion and aging in the U.S. shows the complexity of the issue: spirituality, spiritual faith, religious faith, faith, religion, religiosity, faith in God, religious commitment, religious involvement, are but a few.

What is consistent throughout much of the writing on religion, spirituality, and aging is that a central goal of research is to be able to measure religion and/or spirituality "as a putative antecedent to health outcomes" of people at various stages of life, but particularly for older people (Sloan, et al. 1999:665). The authors of one study, for example, advocate the use of a "spiritual assessment" as part of medical encounters as a means of bringing consideration of a patient's spirituality into the doctor/patient relationship (Anandarajah and Hight 2001). In the "HOPE"[6] assessment discussed by Anandarajah and Hight, physicians are encouraged to ask a series of questions to determine whether a patient is religiously oriented and, if so, how important religion and spirituality are to him or her. Questions such as: "Are you part of a religious community?" "Do you believe in God?" "What kind of relationship do you have with God?" "What aspects of your spirituality or spiritual practices do you find most helpful to you personally?" "Has being sick affected your relationship with God?" are to be asked as part of the process of assessing a patient's religiousness or spirituality (Anandarajah and Hight 2001).

The potential problems with the idea of physicians or other medical personnel giving "spirituality assessments" or assessments of religiousness are extensive. In response to the article by Anandarajah and Hight, Sloan notes the potential ethical problems that can arise. He argues, for example, that in linking religious activity with improved health outcomes, "the physician also implies the converse: that poor health outcomes are associated with insufficient devotion" (Sloan 2001:33). He goes on to point out that by distinguishing patients for whom spirituality and religion are significant aspects of their lives from those for whom they are not, "physicians run the risk of discriminating by encouraging only the former group to engage in religious activity" (Sloan 2001:33). Thus, as he argues, two classes of patients would be created, those who receive the advice and those to whom it is not given. If religious activity is an important adjunct to medical treatment, and the health benefits of religious or spiritual activity significant, should doctors prescribe attendance in church or other forms of religious and spiritual activities?

There is here, I think, a deeper issue, one that is connected to the ethical concern Sloan raises. The concepts of religion and spirituality that are used throughout much of the literature on religion, spirituality, and aging have been largely ethnocentric. This is partially a result of the fact that, for the most part, the studies that have been completed on religion and aging have worked from an "experience-distant" perspective as opposed to an "experience-near" perspective. An experience-distant perspective is one that the observer or researcher uses for the purpose of achieving particular scientific or practical aims, such as determining the relationship between prayer and health. An experience-near perspective is one that someone such as a patient or an elderly person "might himself naturally and effortlessly use to define what he or his fellows see, feel, think, imagine, and so on" (Geertz 1983:57). By emphasizing the experience-distant perspective—the perspective of the researcher—at the exclusion of the experience-near perspective we do not obtain emic interpretations, and thus interpretations generated from within the cultural context of the informant, to be used in constructing etic models and interpretations of religious and spiritual behavior as it relates to aging. The point here is that the study of religion, spirituality, and aging needs to work from the perspective not only of the researcher, but also from the subjectivities of those people being studied. Before determining how religion or spirituality can be assessed or measured and fit into a model of health improvement—if that should be a goal at all—we need to know what these things are from the perspectives of those who think about and practice them.

Thomas and Eisenhandler argue that in order to develop an understanding of religion and spirituality in later life, as well as its potential relationship to health and well-being, social scientists and other scholars need to learn more about the content of religious beliefs, rather than focusing on frequency of prayer, church attendance, or the institutional belief system to which an individual subscribes (Thomas and Eisenhandler 1999:xvii). They go on to suggest the importance of coping with existential issues of human being and the religious question Tillich terms "ultimate concern" (Thomas and Eisenhandler 1999:xxii), which is intimately tied to the existential question of death. I think that this is the right approach, as will become clear shortly, but there remains a problem. Although Thomas and Eisenhandler rightly recognize the importance of individual experience in considering the role of religion and spirituality in the lives of the elderly, they do not point out that experience is structured and interpreted within the framework of culture.

Indeed, when there has been an attempt to define or cope with the issue of the complexity of individual interpretation in conceptualizing religion within gerontology, the results have been largely unsatisfying, in part due to a failure to recognize the importance of culture in how religion is conceptualized and experienced. For example, in the first chapter of his edited volume *Aging, Spirituality, and Religion*, the eminent scholar of religion and aging, Harold Koenig, defines religion in the following way:

> Religion as it is used in this chapter is primarily that based in the Jewish and Christian traditions, monotheistic perspectives that see God as distinct and separate from creation, yet immensely interested in this creation and its future (Koenig 1995:11).

Koenig goes on to indicate that because most Americans are Christians or Jews, this particular "definition" of religion is appropriate, since his study is based in the U.S. The approach Koenig takes underscores the problems related to defining religion in terms of specific sects or denominations. First, Koenig leaves unproblematic Christian and Jewish conceptualizations of "creation" and of "God." The assumption here is that creation and God are uncontested ontological givens rather than polysemous concepts that vary not only among sects, but from person to person even within a single church. One wonders where Unitarian Universalists, who in New England, at least, are often viewed as the most theologically liberal branch of Christianity, would fit into this picture. Furthermore, the "definition" is largely little more than a description of specific beliefs within the Judeo-Christian heritage. There is no concern here about the function of religion, nor about the manner in which individuals variably engage religious beliefs, including those about the nature of their gods. Religion here is treated as a set of beliefs, influenced by doctrinal writings, interpreted in largely uniform ways across sects and denominations.

Indeed, throughout virtually all of the work on religion, spirituality, and aging, religion is equated with the monotheism of Christianity, and to a lesser extent Judaism and Islam, and "God" (always written with a capital "G") is treated as an unproblematic being rather than a concept generated out of various cultural frameworks. Throughout the research on this topic, polytheism is largely ignored. In short, the question of what religion is—its function, its conceptual composition, its relationship to culture—is not explored in the literature, nor are findings from other fields, such as anthropology, that do consider these issues, incorporated into the writings on the topic. If social gerontologists are to develop a better understanding of the relationship between religion, spirituality, and health in old age, they need to begin by trying to understand each of these concepts with reference to the cultures and the experience-near interpretations of the people whose behavior they study.

Having stated this, there remains heuristic value in attempting to explore some of the approaches to a general definition of religion that have been proffered within anthropology and other social sciences. Definitions of religion have often involved reference to the supernatural or to spiritual beings, souls, and deities. In the late 19th Century, E.B. Tylor, in his effort to develop an evolution-based understanding of religious development, presented as a minimum definition of religion, "the belief in Spiritual Beings" (Tylor 1873:424). While this definition has a certain basic appeal, it becomes problematic as one looks at ethnographic research from societies, like Japan, that place very little emphasis on belief as it relates to religious activity. Indeed, as Weber notes, defining religion is fundamentally problematic because religious behaviors are so diverse that understanding can only be achieved by focusing on the subjective experiences and interpretations of those involved, by considering how individuals interpret the meaning of religious behavior (Weber 1963:1).

Problematic as it may be, scholars have frequently endeavored to arrive at some kind of general definition of religion. Some definitions of religion that have been developed in the social sciences have eschewed direct mention of spiritual beings, instead focusing on either the functions or meanings associated with religious and ritual practice. Durkeheim, for example, argues that a "religion is a unified system of beliefs and practices relative to sacred things, that is to say, things set apart and forbidden—beliefs and practice which unite into one single moral community called a Church, all those who adhere to them" (Durkheim 1965 [1915]:62). For Durkheim, the function of religious activity as a collective form of identity articulation is central in understanding the nature of religious action. Through individual and group enactment, religious practice represents the collectivity to its own members, and to outsiders, as a community unified in its common morality. Religion then is in essence one element of the glue—the moral element—that holds a society together.

Geertz's definition of religion as a symbolic system that works to generate moods and motivations and formulate universal conceptualizations of the order of existence that seem inherently factual brings us closer to a workable definition for my purposes here (Geertz 1973). But this definition is open to the critique that it fails to involve reference to the supernatural or spirits and, thus, makes religion difficult to differentiate from political philosophies such as monarchism or democracy (Hicks 1999:11). The basic problem lies in trying to dif-

ferentiate religion from other realms of human activity. How are religious beliefs and behaviors different from political beliefs and behaviors? It is Tillich, although writing within the context of Christian theology, who provides a definition of religion that is most useful
for the discussion I will develop here. Religion for Tillich is defined
simply as ultimate concern. This ultimate concern is something that
moves beyond the realm of particular symbolic systems, particular
ritual activities, and even particular deities (including the Christian
god). Tillich asks the question: What concerns us *unconditionally* or
ultimately? His answer is that which concerns humans ultimately is
"that which determines our being or not-being" (Tillich 1951:14). It
is here, within the framework of contemplating the relationship between being and not-being, and considering that which may have
power over those states, that one encounters religion. Religion is contemplation and expression of human being, as it is continually threat-
ened and preserved, through symbols, deities, rituals, dogmas, and
so on that try to capture and represent that ultimate concern and give
it meaning.

For Tillich, humans are ultimately concerned about their being and
the meaning of that being. This approach to defining religion is particularly helpful for understanding religion as it is practiced in Japan,
because any definition of religion for the Japanese case necessitates
abandoning the idea that religion is necessarily concerned with a capital "G" god or that deities are even the central players in the religious
life. Indeed, Japanese religion centers around the issue of being. More
precisely, Japanese religious practice is most directly associated with
the wellness of being, both for the living and the dead. Ultimate concern in Japan focuses upon the collective well-being of the key spiritual unit in Japanese life—the family—and the entities which give
being meaning—the ancestors. The integration of ultimate concern
into the lives of people occurs through the enactment of ritual, understood as a structure or set of relations among people, living or
dead, and involving sequences of formalized acts and utterances that
are performed in relatively consistent ways (Rappaport 1999:24).

Throughout this book, my focus will center upon the ritual, ceremonial, and ritualistic behaviors of Japanese that structure religious

life. For Japanese, religion is a system of meanings and practices that form what Reader and Tanabe call a "total-care system" that provides for individual and communal needs in both material and spiritual terms throughout the course of one's life (Reader and Tanabe 1998:31). From birth to death and into the afterlife, Japanese engage in a variety of ritual practices variously associated with the institutionalized religions of Shintō and Buddhism that are designed to secure well-being for oneself, one's family, and one's community (company, neighborhood, nation, etc.). Japanese religious practice can be understood as forming something akin to the ways in which people use an HMO, in which they engage in both preventative and curative activities aimed at ensuring health and well-being, which are often conceptualized in terms of success in life and avoidance of medical, physical, or other forms of catastrophe.

Of course, I do not want to simply equate Japanese religious practice and the HMO system in the U.S. through this analogy. Indeed, HMOs in the U.S. are bureaucratic structures that provide services through a capitalist economic system and, thus, are aimed primarily at earning a profit. Because the source of profit lies in the health of their patients, HMOs have a vested interest in maintaining the health and well-being of those patients. While Japanese religious institutions are by no means averse to capitalism—indeed the sale of religious objects to tourists and pilgrims is a major source of income for larger shrines and temples—the goal is certainly not one of profit, thus the analogy has its limits. However, there is a sense in which Japanese religious practice is a systematic approach to ensuring personal and collective well-being, and in this sense there are similarities with the HMO. In Japan, one may enact religious rituals to request help from the Buddhist deity Kannon, the goddess of mercy, to avoid senility and experience a quick and painless death. One may visit a Shintō shrine to petition a deity associated with academic performance for success in college entrance examinations. Or one may have one's new car blessed by a Shintō priest and purchase a talisman (*omamori*) to ensure safe travel. In each case, the activity is focused upon maintaining wellness of being through a system of institutional and non-institutional venues and symbolic resources.

Health and Well-Being

We will return to these themes and explore them in detail later in the book. In presenting religion in the Japanese context in this way, it is necessary to consider what is meant by well-being and health. From an anthropological perspective, health can never be understood as a neutral, biological category or variable (Adelson 2000:3). Health is instead "a complex, dynamic process" rather than a "baseline standard of biomedical or epidemiological normalcy" (Adelson 2000:3). Health is not a universal characteristic of undiseased and non-ill bodies, but is culturally constructed as bodies interact with other bodies and with the social and physical milieu in which they live. In other words, health, like illness, cannot be taken as an *a priori* category of human being that exists as the unproblematic antithesis of unhealth. Nor can it be understood in terms of purely biomedical (positivistic) ideals of biological fitness, presented as an ontological fact of a particular human body without reference to the social conditions in which that body exists. Health is rooted in culturally circumscribed concepts of normalcy and abnormalcy. It is conceptualized in terms of definitions related to what is a normal body, a normal mind, and in relation to gerontology, the normal process of aging; a process often described as "successful aging" and associated with a lack of illness or disease (Rowe and Kahn 1998).

As Adelson argues, the biomedical concept of health permeates and is embodied in the ways in which North Americans define well-being, such that "values such as self-discipline, self-denial, control and will power" are intertwined with concepts of health (Adelson 2000:7). While Japanese are certainly well aware of and often quite oriented towards the biomedical concept of health, this concept is not so thoroughly engaged in structuring how Japanese think about well-being. Instead, well-being, which is closely related to physical and mental health, but also includes broader ideas of success and avoidance of calamity, is interwoven with values of family, self-discipline, and control that are constructed not only in terms of biomedicine, but in terms of social interactions. As will become clear later in the book, a healthy person is one who is not only physically fit, although this certainly enters into the picture, but one who is socially connected. Well-being is not simply a characteristic of an individual, but is a characteristic of the group (particularly the family) to which he or she belongs, thus the individual has a responsibility to engage in activities that will protect and promote that well-being (of which individual health is a part). Religious activities that center upon ancestor veneration and shrine visitations are an important aspect in ensuring collective well-being.

Methods and Writing

Data collection for this book occurred during three trips to Japan in which I conducted ethnographic fieldwork focused largely on understanding Japanese ideas about, and experiences of, the aging process. The first trip, from January of 1995 to August of 1996, took place in a hamlet in northern Japan known as Jōnai in the town of Kanegasaki. I have described this hamlet in detail in the book *Taming Oblivion* (Traphagan 2000a), but I will to some extent add to that description in this volume. A second trip took place for six months in 1998 in the city of Mizusawa, which borders on Kanegasaki. Finally, during the summer of 2000, I spent three months in Akita Prefecture collecting data to compare with and augment the data from Kanegasaki and Mizusawa.

Data were collected through a variety of methods, with a focus on often long and repeated interviews with several key informants. In many cases, I have interviewed all members of a family and I lived within the neighborhoods in Kanegasaki and Mizusawa in which most of my informants lived. Interviews were usually taped, but the content of many informal conversations also contributed considerably to the writing of this volume.

It is important to devote space here to some of the problems inherent in ethnographic research on aging through the technique of participant observation. Participant observation is often presented as one of the hallmarks of cultural anthropology. In ethnography, participant observation is a technique for data collection that is usually described in introductory college text books as consisting of learning a people's culture by direct involvement in their daily lives over long periods of time (Haviland 1999:14). This seems straightforward enough, but it is important to ask what it means to "participate" in a culture. How does one observe as a participant, and what does it mean to be a participant, not simply in an event, conflict, or daily activity, but in a way such that one develops some level of empathy for what it is to be a member of a particular group of people? When one is doing research on the elderly, how can one participate in being old if one is young?

Roger Sanjek discusses a series of interviews he conducted with anthropologists about the nature of fieldwork. At one point he notes that many anthropologists go into the field with the idea of wanting to become "one of the locals" only to give this up when they realize that it is impossible (Sanjek 1990:17). Indeed, anthropologists do not succeed in becoming "locals." They are inevitably researchers attempting to create contexts in which they can learn something about life among the people whom they study. Fieldwork is not a passive activity in which the observer asks questions, writes notes, and then puts them down in fieldnotes later. It is a process in which the ethnographer and his or her informants collaborate in creating contexts of experience that are interpreted by both (Kondo 1990:17). This point is particularly important for the ethnographic study of aging. As a man in his thirties when I did most of the fieldwork for this book, it was simply impossible to adequately share the experience of being 60, or 70, or 90, because I have yet to live through those years of the life course.

This is significant in Japanese society, where age is central in defining the relative position of power and status between and among people. In most cases, I presented something of an anomaly for my informants, particularly during my first long-term fieldwork for my dissertation. My informants were older, wiser, and more experienced than I, and many made this clear to me on several occasions. I was usually referred to as John-*chan*, -*chan* being a diminutive used by an elder towards a younger person (often a child) who is in some way close, but also indicating a power relationship in which the elder holds higher status over the younger. At the same time, during the 1995–96 trip, many were aware that I was affiliated with Tokyo University, which is the most prestigious university in Japan, and sometimes I would be referred to as Traphagan-*sensei*, particularly by people closer to me in age who were meeting me for the first time. The word *sensei* means teacher and is used for those in positions of high status, such as doctors, lawyers, teachers, and college professors. At times, owing to the general ambiguity of my status, people with some knowledge of English would refer to me as "Mr. John", a moniker that brought my wife considerable amusement since it was also the name of a portable toilet company in Pittsburgh.

Throughout each fieldwork experience, I have been involved in a collaborative effort with my informants to find an identity that put them at ease. Researcher, exchange student, husband of a Japanese woman who grew up in Iwate, college professor—all of these have been identities through which I have been interpreted and that I have used as an interpretation of myself to help my informants make sense of my purposes and aims in pressing myself upon their space and into their lives. The one identity that was not negotiated was that of my age. Routinely, my elder informants would bluntly ask my age, and then adjust speech styles and other behaviors accordingly. The identity of elder was one that I could not assume, and I was constantly reminded of this in a multitude of subtle and not-so-subtle ways by my informants during each field trip.

In other words, inasmuch as I could be a participant observer, the one very important aspect of the lives of my informants that I was blocked from participating in was being old. I could not participate in the aches and pains of later life. This was hammered home one day at the completion of a gathering for elderly people at a local meeting hall. All of the participants, including me, were sitting for a very long time in the formal Japanese style of kneeling and sitting on one's legs. When the meeting adjourned, the sounds of bones cracking and popping were ubiquitous, which brought much laughter to the group. While I was able to join in the laughter, I could not participate in the feeling of having those old legs; my legs were numb, but were not creaky.

A great deal of ink has been spent in recent years on the importance of gender in shaping the experience and interactions of the anthropologist with his or her informants. In many contexts, men will be more able to become close to other men and will, thus, be more able to gather intimate details of their lives; the same is often true for women in communicating with female informants. The issue of age has been largely ignored by anthropologists as a limiting factor in data collection. However, it is very important in contexts that place strong emphasis on age-identity as a means of defining social relationships. Japan is such a context and this played an important role in how I went about interacting with my informants and, thus, how I collected data.

The Program

In the following chapters, I will explore the manner in which Japanese people intertwine ideas about religion with those about health and well-being and how this is related to the behavior of older people and to the aging process. Japan is a particularly good context in which to consider how culture is closely tied to the intersection of religious practice and aging, because, as noted above, the basis of Japanese religious activity is quite removed from the doctrinal, faith-based, exclusivist, and belief-oriented tendencies of the focus of most research on this topic—the Judeo-Christian group of religions. Japanese religious activity is related to institutional religious organizations including Buddhist sects, Shintō, and a variety of so-called "new" religions that have arisen in the past 150 years (and that often have tendencies more akin to religious orders in the West in terms of both exclusivity and dependence on some level of doctrine).

Japan is also interesting because Japanese people appear to exhibit a trend towards increased religious activity as they grow older, although it remains unclear as to whether this can be considered an age effect or a cohort effect. Within the gerontological research on religion and aging, a central question has been why people appear to become increasingly involved in religious activity as they grow older. Common answers to this question include the idea that as people grow older, they become increasingly concerned with their own mortality, particularly as they watch people of their own age cohort pass away. As a result, people turn to religious symbols and rituals to cope with the process of aging and dying. An alternative explanation is that people do not actually become increasingly religious, but the current cohort of elderly has always been more religiously active than younger cohorts. Thus, these possibilities for explaining higher levels of religious activities among older people can be attributed to either a cohort effect or an age effect.

When considered with other data, increased belief in the existence of Buddhist deities seems particularly interesting in terms of its relevance for older Japanese, because Buddhism is largely a religion of death and ancestor veneration in Japan. Participation in annual observances related to the dead, in the form of grave visits to make offerings and to clean the grave site, rises from approximately 75 percent for people age 40 to virtually 100 percent for people age 70 and above (Swyngedouw 1993:54). Furthermore, the recent popularity among elderly Japanese, particularly women, of visiting Sudden Death Temples (*pokkuri-dera*)—at which they pray for a sudden, peaceful death devoid of excessive suffering—also suggests a linkage between meanings of religious observances and old age (Wöss 1993:192). Elderly people throughout Japan visit such temples, often as part of excursions organized by Buddhist Lay Associations, Senior Citizens Clubs, or even travel agents (Davis 1992:25). In one survey conducted on reasons worshipers attend sudden death temples, 93 percent stated that it was because they did not wish to become bedridden and a burden on other people. The second most common response (18 percent) was that people did not want to suffer with a prolonged illness like cancer (Wöss 1993:195). Both of these results suggest a connection between religious activities and physical and mental well-being, both for the elderly person and for his/her family. Furthermore, these data suggest that, at least in relation to Buddhist activities, increased participation may be at least partially an age effect connected to concern about individual and familial well-being.

These issues—the manner in which religious ideas and practices are culturally constructed in Japan and the relationship of the elderly to religious practice—are the basis for identifying the theoretical implications of this study. I will argue that rather than generating well-being among the elderly, as is commonly argued to be the case for religiously oriented elders in the U.S., religious participation is a reflection of basic assumptions about interdependence and reciprocity that shape Japanese ideas about human relationships and that the elderly take on the role of caretakers of collective well-being through managing religious ritual performance. I will return to this point at the end of the book and discuss its implications for theoretical work in the study of aging and religion.

Before moving onward, it is necessary to provide some basic details about how I have approached the organization of what follows. In chapter 2, I will diverge from the theoretical issues I have explored in this chapter and focus on ethnographic description of the context in which research for this book took place. The purpose of chapter 2 is to provide a detailed look at the context in which older people in rural Japan experience their later years. I will argue that the difficulties of old age associated with isolation and alienation are neither limited to large urban areas, nor to elders living apart from younger family members. I will present several forms of data that show some of the difficulties contemporary elders living in rural areas experience and also explore how growing old is closely intertwined with institutional structures related to provision of health care. Following this, in chapter 3, I will discuss Japanese conceptualizations of illness and health or well-being and how these are closely related to ideas about the importance of social interaction in generating health and well-being. Chapters 4 and 5 focus on Japanese religious practice in terms of the concept of concern and argue that through private and public forms of religious participation, Japanese people are enacting concern about the well-being of individuals, families, and communities. At the center of this enactment of concern are the elderly, who are caretakers of individual and collective concern. In chapter 6, I will consider the role of ancestors in the world of the living, and discuss dreams that are interpreted as signs of concern on the part of the ancestors. This chapter will focus on the importance of older women in conveying ancestral concern to the world of the living, a practice that is closely related to the association of the feminine with caregiving in the Japanese context. Finally, in chapter 7, I will return to some of the themes raised in this chapter and provide concluding thoughts on the nature of the relationship between religious activity, well-being, and aging in Japan and discuss the implications of the study in terms of the manner in which medical anthropology can inform theoretical work in gerontology that deals with the study of religion and aging.

Chapter 2

Aging and Anomie in Rural Japan

In this neighborhood, virtually everyone is living in a one-gen-
eration elderly household. Almost all of the children around
here have left to go elsewhere. There are a lot of people around
my age whose children have moved away.

— 65 year-old man living in Mizusawa

Rural Japan often is symbolically represented as a place removed
from the urban anomie and industrial dehumanization associated
with metropolitan areas such as Tokyo. In the Japanese news media
and in popular television shows, rural people are presented as living
closer to a pure Japanese lifestyle that embodies traditional values of
community and family. This pattern is nothing new, having been
common for much of the 20th Century, during which rural Japan has
often been associated with an authentic, traditional Japan in many
ways apart from, and superior to, the urban and modern (cf.
Tamanoi 1998 and Creighton 1997). Older people in rural areas are
more likely to live in multi-generation households than those living
in cities. Thus, there is an image that more rural elderly live a life that
at least approximates the ideal presented in rhetoric related to a good
life in old age: that is, co-residence or close proximity to one's eldest
child (particularly one's eldest son), his or her spouse, and their children. Perhaps like so many romanticized representations, ideals about
elder life in *inaka*, the word typically used to refer to less urban areas,

are often far removed from the realities of loneliness and distance from loved ones that, in fact, characterize the experiences of many like the man quoted at the beginning of this chapter.

In areas like Tōhoku, urban anomie may be replaced by a rural anomie as older people experience alienation from younger family members with whom they live or the loneliness of life amidst a sprawling farmhouse in which no one else resides. In many cases, older people living in rural areas view themselves as isolated from contemporary society. Elderly often describe themselves as *furui,* meaning old and outdated or obsolete. There are impediments to interacting with younger family members, the most commonly identified being differences in values among young and old and sometimes even differences in dialect.

The Tōhoku dialect is particularly well-known throughout Japan for its divergence from the standard Japanese used on television and taught in school. For example, the word for "yes" in standard Japanese is *"hai",* while in some Tōhoku dialects, including the one used around Kanegasaki and Mizusawa, the word normally used is *"ndanda."* In standard Japanese, one might say *"ikimasen ka"* which means "shall we not go?" while in Kanegasaki one would possibly say *"ikanegasu ka,"* although the standard form is also used. Although older people are generally able to understand both standard Japanese and their local dialect, they often are not able to produce the standard dialect, thus making communication with grandchildren, in particular, difficult, since younger people often do not have command of the local dialect. Lamenting this social distancing, one woman in her seventies stated that she doubted that her grandchildren understood more than 30 or 40 percent of what she said to them.

While dialect differences do inhibit communication and interaction among young and old, people also often comment that values between younger and older generations are so different as to make mutual understanding almost impossible. This is perceived as a central reason why co-residence, which as I will discuss below is often represented as a desirable residential arrangement particularly for grandparents and grandchildren, can generate stress and conflict between the middle and elder generations. For example, Torisawa Michiko, who was in her late thirties when we talked, spoke in detail about the differences she perceived in the values of younger and elder generations and how these differences made co-residence between the two difficult (this case is also discussed in Traphagan 2003a, Case 4):

> **Torisawa:** The main problem [of co-residing] is that there are totally different values between young and old. Because the values [*kachikan*] are different, it is impossible for us to fully adjust to each other. The only way to deal with my father-in-law is to remain silent and not talk to him or give opinions. If I say nothing, it is o.k. I can't really talk to my in-laws. I don't like the way in which my father-in-law thinks he is *erai* [high status] and the master of the entire household.
> **JWT:** What are the differences in values between younger and older people?
> **Torisawa:** First, old people don't have any sense of enjoyment in their lives. They only work and view any form of leisure or recreation as a waste of time. They don't do things like enjoying eating nice food. They just eat to live and have no interest in things like good food or the like. They just work and sleep, but they do not do anything else. Second, we don't agree on what is waste. Building a new house on the same land or living in Mizusawa is a waste of money to them, so we shouldn't do it. There is no concept of the need for separate living space or privacy. Third, parents think that children are always children and are, therefore, always under the control of the parents. There is no concept that, having become an adult, you have independence and have lost the situation of being under your parents' control. We are actively trying to socialize our children not to think this way and are trying to keep them away from the grandparents in terms of this sort of thing so that they will not grow up to think that they have to do what their parents say.

Another woman in her late thirties, who was not co-residing with her in-laws but who had experienced co-residence with them for more than a year, went as far as to comment that: "In Japan, children are the belongings of their parents. They are pets [*shoyūdobutsu*]."

For both young and old Japanese living in rural areas, at least, there is a clear perception of a very wide generation gap that makes communication and living in close proximity difficult. As we see in Torisawa's narrative, concern over vastly different values is significant enough that the younger couple has made conscious efforts to socialize and educate their children in a manner distinct from that which they experienced while growing up. They want their children to have different expectations about what they can do and the degree to which they must follow the path set by their parents.

I will return to Torisawa's narrative later in the chapter. Prior to that, however, I want to devote some attention to exploring perceptions about a generation gap that at times appears so wide, at least from an outsider's perspective, that it is as though there are two distinct cultures co-existing in the same physical and temporal space. Among older Japanese, perceptions about the depth of this generation gap are closely related to feelings of isolation. As one woman explained while discussing the difficulties people face in old age in Mizusawa:

> Although in *inaka* there are more people living in multi-generation families [than in the cities], even if there is an image of the household as *nigiyaka* [lively or bustling], there are many who live in solitude [*kodoku*]. I think that this kind of solitude or isolation is part of the reason that suicide is common among the elderly [in rural areas]. Even if the children and grandchildren are around, there are various things that interfere with the connection between the elderly and others.

Indeed, suicide among the elderly, particularly in rural areas where the proportion of elderly in the population is generally higher than in the cities, is a serious problem; one that differentiates the Japanese experience of modernity and postmodernity from that of most other industrial societies.[1] In 2000, according to Ministry of Health, Labor, and Welfare statistics, the suicide rate for people over 90 was 47.8 per 100,000 nationally. For those between 85 and 89, the rate was 47.1, and for those between 80 and 84 it was 40.7. By contrast, the rate for people in their twenties and thirties was approximately 20 in 2000 (Nakata 2002). Satomi Kurosu notes that sociological studies of suicide among the elderly outside Japan have repeatedly shown that urban, industrialized areas in which there has been some degree of breakdown in social integration generally have higher elder suicide rates than rural areas (Kurosu 1991:604). She notes that Japan has been one of the few locales (others are Greece and California) in which suicide rates were found to be lower in urban than in rural areas. Drawing on data from the early 1980's, Kurosu shows that during that period the suicide rates for prefectures with low-density population exceeded 120, while those for high-density areas have consistently registered rates below 80, working from an index of 100 (1991:604).

This trend continues into the present. Figure 2.1 shows the prevalence rates of suicides by age group for Iwate Prefecture in 1990 and 1995 (suicides as a proportion of all deaths for each age group). It is clear that from the mid-60's suicides represent an increasing proportion of total deaths. Figure 2.2 shows the proportion of deaths classified as suicides by selected Tōhoku prefectures and for Japan for the year 2000. Both Akita and Iwate prefectures had rates considerably higher than Japan as a whole, as well as higher than Tokyo and Miyagi Prefecture, in which the regional center of Sendai, with a population of about 1 million people, is located. In Akita, 457 people committed suicide in 2000, representing 3.80 percent of the total deaths; in Iwate these numbers were 454 suicides and 3.63 percent. By contrast, in large urban areas, the proportion of deaths attributed to suicide was generally lower. In Tokyo 3.32 percent of deaths were attributed to suicide, in Miyagi Prefecture 316 percent, and in Fukushima the proportion was only 2.68 percent. It is important to avoid drawing too much of a conclusion from these numbers—some rural prefectures, such as Yamagata, also located in Tōhoku, show proportions that are among the lower numbers. However, it is clear that there is a general tendency for suicide rates to be higher in rural than in urban areas, particularly when considering the elderly.

This pattern of higher suicide rates in rural areas has developed over the past fifty years. For example, in 1955, there were approximately 275 suicides in Akita Prefecture, ranking it 39th out of 48 prefectures in the nation as a whole when the number of suicides is taken

Figure 2.1 Prevalence Rate of Suicides by Age Group for Iwate Prefecture, 1990 and 1995

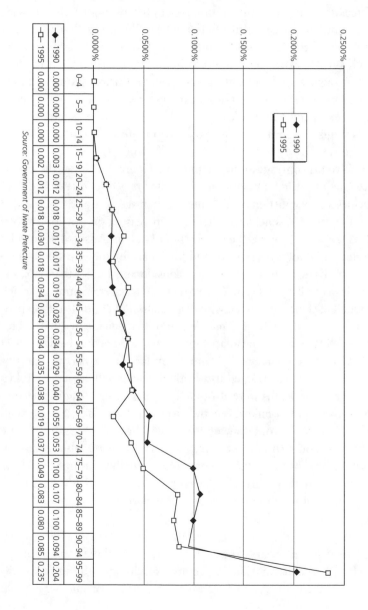

Source: Government of Iwate Prefecture

Figure 2.2 Proportion of Total Deaths Classified as Suicide for 2000

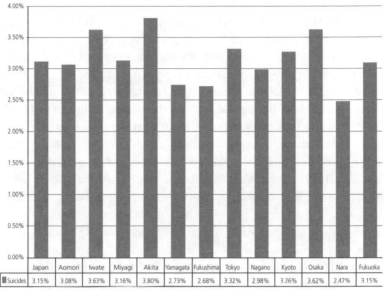

	Japan	Aomori	Iwate	Miyagi	Akita	Yamagata	Fukushima	Tokyo	Nagano	Kyoto	Osaka	Nara	Fukuoka
■ Suicides	3.15%	3.08%	3.63%	3.16%	3.80%	2.73%	2.68%	3.32%	2.98%	3.26%	3.62%	2.47%	3.15%

Source: Japan Statistical Yearbook, Statistics Bureau, Ministry of Public Management, Home Affairs, Posts and Telecommunications
(http://www.stat.go.jp/english/data/nenkan/zuhyou/b1919000.xls)

as a proportion of total population. By 1970, Akita had moved into the top ten prefectures for suicides and from 1985 until the present the prefecture has consistently ranked number one or two in the nation (Asahi Shinbun Atkia Shikyoku 2000:5) and has ranked number one in the nation for six consecutive years at the time of this writing (Nakata 2002).[2]

My purpose here is not to delve into a detailed discussion of suicide among rural elderly. Rather, it is to point out the depth of despair some rural elders reach. The question of why this occurs, when many elders in rural areas live amidst the idealized mutli-generation family, raises an important question: Is there a relationship between the Japanese family system and alienation among rural elders? The answer, I think, is yes. But before addressing this, it is necessary to devote more attention to how Japanese people conceptualize the family.

Social Networks: Family and Friends

The family, and more specifically the stem-family system, has been a central theme in research on Japanese culture both by Japanese and non-native social scientists and has occupied an important place in anthropological writing on Japan (Aruga 1954; Brown 1968, 1980; Hamabata 1990; Ochiai 1997; Traphagan 2000b). There has been considerable debate concerning the nature of the stem-family (*ie* in Japanese), focusing on whether it is primarily to be understood as an economic unit centered around a particular occupation (Befu 1963; Nakane 1967) or a family and residential unit organized around affective bonds among its members. (Brown 1966; Lebra 1993, Long 1987; Traphagan 2000b) Both perspectives have merit, but as the nuclear family has become a more common living arrangement in Japan since the end of World War II, it seems to be clear that while the economic elements of the stem-family are important to recognize, the contents of familial relations within the stem-family are social and affective and can operate devoid of any economic or occupational center around which a given stem-family may be organized (Brown 1968). Although the term *kazoku* is often used for the immediate, nuclear family, even individuals living in nuclear family arrangements distant from each other will often still use the term *ie* to describe their extended families and will usually describe individuals in terms of the social position within the stem-family that he or she holds, such as eldest son, eldest daughter, head of household, and so on.

The centrality of the stem-family system as a general form of family organization dates back to 1898, when the Meiji Civil Code extended the family system of the samurai class to the entire population, requiring that everyone be registered as part of a stem-family (Lock 1993:87). The term used to identify the stem-family, *ie*, involves a complex of conceptual and physical expressions that include the family, the household (understood as a unit of residence that may include both kin and non-kin such as servants), and the house itself. Writing in the 1930's Embree described a farmer's household, in particular, in terms that continue to be relevant in contemporary society:

Here the entire household lives together; here dwell the spirits of the ancestors in the Buddhist alcove (*butsudan*); and here, in some smoke blackened corner of the kitchen, are the homely deities of good fortune, Ebisusan and Daikokusan. Here also are the household gods who look after the kitchen, the well, and the toilet, respectively (Embree 1964 [1939]:89).

While the smoke blackened corner of the kitchen is gone from modern farmhouses, the ancestors and household gods (such as Suijin, the deity of the well) often continue to reside alongside the living as part of the household. Indeed, the stem-family is not limited in time to the present, but represents a historically defined center of continuity for, and including, a lineally descended group of preferably blood-related living and dead, inherited and acquired property, and in some cases a specific occupation that is passed down over generations, although non-consanguineal relations may also be part of the stem-family, such as in the case of adoption (Traphagan 2000a). Continuity is maintained via descent reckoned within the framework of a family system that promotes male primogeniture and succession to the headship of the household. Succession is usually determined patrilineally, with either the eldest or another son in the event that the eldest is unwilling or unable to succeed, taking over the household headship and the headship of the family farm or business (if these exist). In the absence of competent and willing male successors, another male may be adopted into the household to take the role of successor (this person is known as *mukoyōshi*). In the past, this often involved adoption of a cousin, but in contemporary society it is likely to be simply a man who is willing to give up his family name and enter into his wife's family register (*koseki*). It is important to recognize that there are exceptions to this tendency, as Yoshida (1997) shows in his study of matrifocal household businesses (inns) in a hot spring town where transfers of property and the family business are passed along female lines.

This system of succession and inheritance is important for understanding aging in contemporary Japanese society, because older Japanese were socialized early in life to expect an old-age in which a male child and that child's spouse and children would co-reside, providing company and, if need be, care as time went on. Akiko Hashimoto (1996) notes that a degree of dependency by elders upon their children is both legitimate and in some respects expected in Japan. This legitimized dependency contributes to the idea among both young and old that filial piety is often best represented through co-residence, although the interpretation of this as positive or negative varies considerably from one person to another. Indeed, Kiefer notes that for the older Japanese living in a retirement community that he and Kinoshita studied, the decision to move into the retirement community represented a kind of behavior that was viewed as in some ways deviant because it rejected dependence upon children for care and formed a "kind of rejection of traditional attitudes about the role of the elderly in family and community" (Kiefer 1999:201, see also Kinoshita and Kiefer 1992).

The persistence of the stem-family as an ideal of family living patterns intensifies the social distancing older people feel in rural areas. They may be unable to attain the type of old age they expected—being forced to live alone or only with a spouse because their children have moved away to other parts of Japan, unable or unwilling to return due to work and the responsibilities of their own nuclear families. Loneliness and isolation are often ascribed to older people who are living alone and this situation is often blamed upon changes in Japanese family structure. When I asked Sakamoto Hiroshi, a man in his sixties when we talked, about why suicide rates for elders in Japan are high, he placed the blame directly on a shift towards the nuclear family structure (*kaku kazoku*):

> There are at least two reasons [why suicide is high among the elderly] in my opinion. First, the movement toward a nuclear family has created a situation in which old people feel out of place. They were educated in a different set of ideals about how the family should be and they feel that they cannot fit into the current family structure. In the past old people had a lot of friends in the neighborhood and had good networks of people upon whom they could de-

pend. This situation has disappeared in the modern world. Old people feel nostalgic [*natsukashii*] for the past and do not feel that they meet with the way the current culture is. Therefore, because they feel out of place, they feel that there is no point in living. Second, when sick, people used to help each other throughout the neighborhood, but this is no longer the case. If one doesn't have friends around then one may not want to live. Finally, I think differences in wealth contribute to suicide. If a person looks around and sees that other people have better housing and more money and live with their children and grandchildren, they become lonely and sad. This sadness of life can lead to suicide among the elderly. Others have what they don't have and they decide that there is no reason to live. I think that this is particularly common among the elderly living alone.

The extent to which Sakamoto's interpretation of the reasons behind high rates of elder suicide represents the actual state of affairs is open to question. As I have shown elsewhere (Traphagan 2000a), the lack of co-resident family members has in some cases led to an increased dependence upon age peers for social support and the presence of Old Persons Clubs (*rōjin kurabu*) in most neighborhoods provides a clear context in which older people can regularly interact with friends and acquaintances of their own age. Furthermore, the nuclearization of the family does not necessarily mean that the elderly are dramatically distanced from their children and grandchildren. It is common for a child and his or her nuclear family to live very close to his or her parents, even to the extent of living in separate living quarters within the same building with the elder generation.

However, from an emic perspective, Sakamoto's views are indicative of a tendency among older people to interpret the high suicide rate and other expressions of anomie among the elderly as being connected to social change in the form of a shift from a three-generation family structure to a nuclear family and to an associated increase in isolation and alienation of older people from both their own families and from their age peers. Sakamoto sees contemporary society as inherently alienating because changing values and conditions have made people less dependent upon each other than they were in the past. Whereas in the past old people could depend upon both family and age peers in times of need, now they do not have either to depend upon easily. In other words, from Sakamoto's perspective along with a change in family structure has come a loss of networks among elder age peers and this has increased the isolation and loneliness of older people.

Government services for the elderly, some of which are designed to create context for older people to interact with their age peers and reduce some of the difficulties that arise with isolation, have grown since the inception of the long-term care insurance program (*kaigo hoken*) in 2000. In Kanegasaki, for example, there are twenty home helpers, a number that has doubled in the past five years, who visit households in which there are elder couples, elders living alone, or in which an individual is bedfast or experiencing significant impairments that require regular attention. There are also food delivery services, help with house repairs, "snow busters" who help with shoveling snow, and various informational meetings and group activities such as "*furiai*" (in touch) hiking to bring people with disabilities together for activities. Figure 2.3 shows the front page from a pamphlet for services available to townspeople. The brochure describes not only services for care recipients, but also services for care providers, such as the *kaigosha rifuresshu* (literally, "nursing provider refresh," although in terms of meaning this is best translated as "care provider refresh" as it is intended for family care providers rather than nursing care professionals) program that gives opportunities for people who are providing care to do physical activities aimed at refreshing the body. The pamphlet describes a "Community Welfare Enterprise for Resident Participation" and indicates that the town will endeavor to provide a range of services that involve volunteer support. And on the top of page one of the brochure it reads "*fureai, sasaeai, manabiai, mitomeai*" which mean touch or contact, support, learn, and recognize, respectively. This slogan is presented as something of a pun in which the "*ai*" portion of each word uses the character for love (the last two terms are invented rather than regular Japanese words). By emphasizing the notion of

Figure 2.3 Social Services pamphlet from Kanegasaki

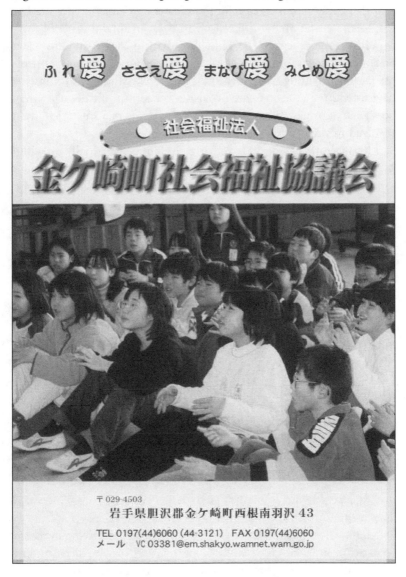

love, the town is attempting to encourage people to connect with each other and to support those in need through volunteer service.

In this sense the brochure and many of the town services provided for elder care (as well as care for the disabled in general, see Traphagan forthcoming a) are directed, at least ostensibly, toward the aim of addressing precisely the kind of isolation and distancing that Sakamoto reflects upon. An emphasis on encouraging people to volunteer for providing care provision is one way that town governments have attempted to center care provision on communities rather than on the government. Many such brochures show pictures of children involved in various types of care-related activities.

Although many elders view change in family as causally linked to isolation and alienation leading to dependence upon government services, it would be a mistake to assume that simple residence within the multi-generation context is a solution to the problem of alienation that Sakamoto attributes to nuclear families. As noted above, an older person may live within the idealized multi-generation family, only to find it difficult to interact or communicate with younger members of the household, a result of both changes in dialect and changes in values. In a discussion with the Woman's Association in the neighborhood in Mizusawa where I lived, I asked the women, all of whom were in their fifties or above, about their experiences in living in multi-generation households. One woman summed up the attitudes of these women well when she stated:

> I often don't feel that I can talk directly to my son because I have to think about it going to his wife, as well. She is sort of in between us and therefore I am forced to hold back. I can't talk from my heart [*kokoro kara*] because his wife is there and if she disagrees with what I think it will turn into a fight [*kenka suru*].

Older people living in rural Japan often experience isolation and alienation both from family members and from the larger society in which they live. While there are certainly happy elders living in multi-generation households, as well as happy elders living alone (many older widows told me that they were in the happiest time of their lives because for the first time they had freedom from caring for others), the broad perception about old age is that changes in family structure, along with broader social change, have created impediments to the experience of a happy old age.

Aging in the Tōhoku Region and Japan

Given the above discussion on the isolation of older people in rural areas, it is important to present a more general look at population aging as it is expressed in the Tōhoku region and Japan nationally. As of 2002, approximately 18 percent of the Japanese population was over the age of 65. This proportion of the population is among the highest in the world, but more striking than the present population distribution are the projections for the aging of the Japanese population in the future. By 2015, the country will have reached a point where 25 percent of the population is over the age of 65; by 2050 it is projected that slightly under one-third of the population will be over 65 (Sōmuchō 2000:41). By comparison to other societies, Japan has reached a condition in which its population could be considered aged (more than 14 percent over the age of 65) with extreme rapidity. In France it required 130 years for the population to shift from seven percent over the age of 65 to 14 percent, in the United Kingdom it took 45 years, and in the U.S. it will take about 70 years for the same transition to occur. In Japan this transition occurred over a period of 25 years from 1970 to 1995 (Kinoshita and Kiefer 1992:42).

The causes behind these demographic trends involve a complex of factors related to low fertility, increased longevity, and, in rural areas, out-migration of young people. During the 1950's Japan experienced a rapid transition in fertility and mortality. In 1947 the total fertility rate (TFR), the average number of children born to a woman over the course of her lifetime, in Japan was 4.54 (by comparison, the TFR for 1925 was 5.11 and for 1937 was 4.37). By 1960, this rate had dropped to 2.0, where it remained relatively stable hovering around replacement level (2.1) until the mid 1970's. In 1975, the total fertility rate dropped below 2.0 (it reached 1.91) and it has not risen above that level since.[3] Although household size continued to decline during this time, more important for the total fertility rate was the fact that more women were choosing not to have children. As Raymo has pointed out, this period is marked by an increase in the proportion of unmarried women in their 20s and early 30s (Raymo 1998:1023).

The decline of the total fertility rate has become an alarming issue for government officials and is annually a major news story. According to the Management and Coordination Agency of the Japanese Ministry of Health and Welfare, as of 2000, the total fertility rate in Japan stood at approximately 1.36 children per woman over the life course. The declining birth rate has been considered serious enough that in July of 2003, the National Diet approved pro-natalist legislation that requires local and national governments to develop programs to encourage birth and calls for fertility treatment support and improvements in child-care services (Asahi Shinbun 2003). Low fertility alone, however, does not account for the rapid aging of the Japanese population, particularly in rural areas. Over the same period, the Japanese have experienced steady reductions in mortality, such that the country has the world's highest life expectancy at birth of 84.60 years for women and 77.72 years for men as of 2000.[4]

In areas removed from metropolitan centers, changes in population structure as a result of decreased fertility and mortality have been exacerbated by long periods of rural-to-urban migration, which, despite having diminished over the past twenty years, continue to drain younger individuals from local populations. Demographic researchers in Japan have pointed out that rural-to-urban migration was the predominant form of population movement until the 1970s. Changes in both legal and political attributes of Japanese society contributed to a significant outflow of people from rural to urban areas following World War II. This pattern began to change in the 1970's when net migration into major metropolitan centers began to decline significantly, particularly following the "oil shock" of 1973, when OPEC (Organization of Oil Exporting Countries) restricted the production of oil and increased prices following the start of the fourth Arab-Israeli War (Liaw 1992:321). After the oil shock, prefectures neighboring major cities began to experience population growth as a result of the so-called "J-turn" pattern of migration in which people began to

Table 2.1 Net-migration for the six prefectures that
comprise the Tōhoku Region, 1980–2001.

Net Migration (- net loss)				
	1980	1990	1995	2000	2001
Aomori	-5,152	-11,007	-695	-2,329	-2,974
Iwate	-4,679	-5,012	-469	-2,222	-3,568
Miyagi	4,164	4,893	7,112	-731	-2,308
Akita	-5,092	-5,066	-1,743	-3,068	-3,137
Yamagata	-3,016	-3,878	-646	-1,734	-3,456
Fukushima	-4,536	-2,235	272	-3,412	-5,782
Average	**-3,052**	**-3,718**	**639**	**-2,249**	**-3,538**

Source: *Japan Statistical Yearbook, Statistics Bureau, Ministry of Public Management,*
Home Affairs, Posts and Telecommunications
(http://www.stat.go.jp/english/data/nenkan/zuhyou/b0230000.xls), see also Sōmuchō 1998.

move out from urban centers to find more affordable housing and less congested environments (Fukurai 1991:41).

During the mid 1980's, there was a brief period during which Tokyo experienced a net gain in population from migration, but this rapidly returned to a pattern of net population loss. By comparison, the Tōhoku region experienced a growth in net losses due to migration from the late 1970's to the late 1980's. As is evident in Table 2.1, as of 1980 the average population loss for the six prefectures that comprise the Tōhoku region was 3,052 and this number increased to 3,718 in 1990. During the mid 1990s, there was a brief period in which net loss due to migration in several Tōhoku prefectures approached zero, with an average gain of 639 in 1995 for the prefectures in Tōhoku, although most of this was the result of a major increase in migration to Miyagi Prefecture where the regional urban center, Sendai (with a population of slightly under one million), is located. By 2001, the average loss for the prefectures in Tōhoku had returned to a level similar to that of 1990, with an average net loss of 3,538.

It is clear that net population loss due to migration, particularly rural-to-urban migration, remains a major feature of the demographic landscape in Tōhoku, particularly when considering people in their late teens and early twenties. It is a common pattern for young women and men who are not expected to succeed to the household headship to move to Tokyo for education and to find work. Finding work in rural areas can be difficult, and the poor national economy has been reflected locally in the closing of numerous businesses or the relocation of businesses away from downtown districts that are difficult to access by car. In the summer of 2002, for example, there were fifteen businesses along the main street of Mizusawa that had closed or moved, thus leaving vacant space, and one large department store that occupied a five-story building had been demolished and was being replaced in the summer of 2003 by a new building for a local bank that was moving from its location on another part of the main street.

In addition to the rapid aging of the Japanese population, residence patterns have also been changing. Figure 2.4 shows the shift in residence patterns from 1980 to 2000. The proportion of the elderly population (those over 65) either living alone or with a spouse only has been on the increase for several years, moving from 10.84 percent to 20.15 percent of the elderly population living alone and 15.67 percent to 26.43 percent living only with a spouse. Over the same period of time the percentage of elders living in three-generation households has dropped from 40.26 percent to 20.86 percent. Clearly, as noted earlier, the traditional three-generation household (parents, married child and their children) is becoming significantly less typical of the living situation of older Japanese, even while the preference for living with a child remains an important feature of the social landscape from an ideological perspective. However, this does not necessarily mean that multi-generation families are simply disappearing. It is very common to find households in which there are two adult generations without children. Often, the younger generation returns to live with the elder generation after the son has retired following a career in another part of Japan. In these cases, while the household consists of two generations, both generations are typically over the age of sixty, thus creating a situation in which one finds two-generation elder households.

It is important to recognize that, although commonly cited as an indication of the breakdown of the traditional Japanese family structure, data such as these can be misleading. While it is clear that

Figure 2.4 Elder Residence Patterns 1980–2000

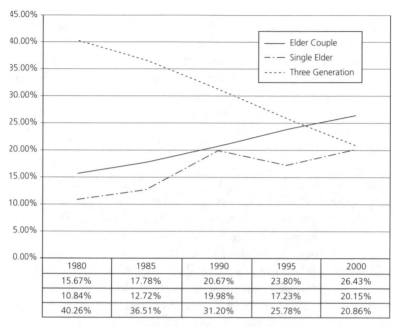

	1980	1985	1990	1995	2000
	15.67%	17.78%	20.67%	23.80%	26.43%
	10.84%	12.72%	19.98%	17.23%	20.15%
	40.26%	36.51%	31.20%	25.78%	20.86%

Source: Statistical Survey Department, Statistics Bureau, Ministry of Public Management, Home Affairs, Posts and Telecommunications
(http://www.stat.go.jp/english/data/nenkan/zuhyou/b0219000.xls)

fewer elderly are living in the same household with their children, alternative patterns of living have developed that still allow for elders to live in close proximity to their children and grandchildren. Perhaps most notable is the *nisetai jūtaku*, as described by Naomi Brown, in which multiple generations live in the same building, while maintaining separate living quarters. Usually, the elder generation lives on the ground floor while the younger generations live on the upper floor of the house. In many cases, the upper-floor living quarters may consist of the conjugal family including children, but it is not uncommon for this generation to only include the son and his wife, their adult children having established their own households. Both sections of the house have separate kitchen and bath facilities, allowing both households to retain privacy while also permitting regular contact among generations and close proximity should the need for elder care arise (see N. Brown 2003).

In other cases, successor children choose to live near, but not with their parents. A common feature of the landscape in rural areas has become the construction of separate houses for the younger and older generations on the same land, forming a compound co-residence situation, rather than co-residence in the same structure. Bernstein (1983) notes this pattern in her work during the 1970's in rural Japan. Young couples would, after a few years living with the husband's parents, move to a separate and smaller dwelling attached to or slightly removed from the main house. This afforded greater privacy for the young couple, and probably took some of the burden off of the daughter-in-law, of whom was expected much by her mother-in-law.

In the case of the family with whom Bernstein lived, the grandmother lived across the street while often eating with the rest of the family in the main house (Bernstein 1983:4–12). Initially, the young married couple had lived in the smaller house while having daily involvement in the life of the main house, in part to retain a degree of privacy, but traded with the grandmother as the young family grew. While the pattern of building a separate house on the same land in order to separate the generations continues to be important in rural areas, reasons behind this living arrangement seem quite different from those described by Bernstein. For example, Matsumoto Yoko was in her mid-thirties when she agreed to move from an apartment in a major city to live with her in-laws in Kanegasaki, with the stipulation that a separate house be built for her nuclear family.[5]

> **JWT:** When you married your husband, did you know that he would become the successor in the household and return to live in this area?
> **Matsumoto:** No, I didn't know [laughs]! I never expected it. My husband is the third son, but his elder brothers have both married and live in Tokyo. They both married women who are only children, so there is no chance that they will return—nor do they want to return. This situation has left it on my husband to be the successor. If I knew that he was

going to become the successor and we would have to live
with his parents, I don't think I would have married him.
JWT: What were things like at the time your husband returned [from Kanegasaki] to Yokohama?
Matsumoto: We fought a great deal and I was very troubled
[*kenka shimashita, nayamimashita*)]. We had also had fights
about returning to live with his parents when we were in
Yokohama together. I said to my husband, "You are being
more concerned about the lives of your parents than you are
of your own family." I thought at the time about not coming
back at all and divorcing him as a result of his behavior.
JWT: Why did you build a separate house when your in-laws
have such a large house?
Matsumoto: It was one of the conditions of moving here. I
told my husband that I would not return unless we built a separate house to live in. My in-laws did not oppose the idea of
building a separate house, which was good. They understood
that we would not return unless the separate house was built.
JWT: Why was it important to have a separate house?
Matsumoto: I was concerned about a variety of things and
wanted privacy. I felt that there would be a great deal of conflict between myself and my mother-in-law if we lived in the
same house. A lot of old people badmouth their daughter-in-
law [*yome*]. The mothers-in-law want the *yome* to go out and
do some sort of work at a job while grandma takes care of the
children. If the *yome* doesn't want to do this, then there is
conflict because the mother-in-law thinks the *yome* should be
bringing in income. I think this is related to concerns older
people have about the values of younger people. The mothers-in-law try to take control over the grandchildren in order
to raise them to behave and think in a way that they consider
to show *oya kōkō* [filial piety]. It is a power struggle over the
raising of the children and to some extent the mother-in-law
has the upper hand because it is her family and the *yome* is es-
sentially an outsider. All of the younger *yome* around here
want to raise their own children, but the mothers-in-law are

strong on trying to get the *yome* to go out and leave the children to them. This creates a lot of stress between the *yome* and mother-in-law. It seems as though mothers-in-law want to take away the grandchildren from the *yome* [*obaachan ga torechau kanji suru*]. The younger women around here say that they might as well go off and get their own apartment because they have no role in raising their children. And the husband won't say anything; if the *yome* complains, the husband just defends the *ie* and his parents. It is very hard to live together.

Matsumoto's situation should not be seen as an isolated case. Another woman, Torisawa, mentioned previously in relation to tensions in values between young and old, had agreed to move from her house in a major metropolitan area to the Mizusawa area only on the condition that a separate house be built. She was concerned about being able to maintain privacy for her children. Torisawa lives with her husband amidst wide expanses of rice paddies on a plot of land where her husband's family has lived for several generations. Approximately three years prior to our conversation, they had built a new house separate from Mr. Torisawa's parents' house. The contrast between the two buildings is stark, with the elder generation's house being an old, rectangular farmhouse with a dingy exterior, and the younger generation's house a modern, white house constructed in a contemporary design that is common throughout the area. The compound is rather spacious and the houses are separated by about 20 meters. The couple co-reside with their ten-year-old daughter and five-year-old son, while Mr. Torisawa's parents and grandfather live in the older building. Thus, there are four generations on the compound, the elder two living in one house and the younger two living in the other.

The couple met in Chiba, a large metropolitan area that is part of the Tokyo metropolis, while he was assigned there by the construction company for which he worked. Eventually, he felt pressured as the eldest son to return to live in his natal home and care for his parents as they grew older. At the time they returned, Mr. Torisawa's grandmother had been bed-ridden for about 15 years. She died not long after their return and, although Mr. Torisawa stated that he did not return specifically for the purpose of caring for his grandmother, concern over filial responsibility and providing care was central in the decision. His most serious concern was his mother, who had been taking care of his grandmother for the entire 15 year period of convalescence. According to Torisawa, she had become very tired and was having difficulties managing all the work required in providing care and taking care of the home, so he decided it was time to return.

The family did not return directly, but first spent time in Sendai, a city of about a million people, and then Mizusawa, before returning to his natal home. The reason for this, they stated, was to allow Mrs. Torisawa to experience a gradual shift from urban to rural life. Thus they calculated a strategy for the return to his natal home: "Because my wife grew up in a large city [Chiba], I didn't think she would easily adjust to life in *inaka*, so I thought that it would take some time to adjust. Therefore, we thought it would be good to start in a city."

The couple consulted with each other quite a bit about the process of return and agreed that a gradual return was needed. They also decided that, as Mr. Torisawa put it:

In order for my wife to come to understand the thinking and lifestyle of my parents and a farm family, she would need time and also for my parents to come to understand her, they would need time. I felt that this was absolutely necessary. The thinking pattern of an old farm family is very different [from city families] and we thought it would be impossible for them to live together. For this reason when we finally decided to return, we felt that it would be necessary to build a house of our own. My father opposed this. He wanted everyone to live in the same house and thought that with such a big house [about 540 square meters] it was a total waste to build another house right next to them. But I felt that there was no chance that our family's lifestyle would work with my parents' lifestyle.

Eventually, the elder generation came to understand that this was going to be the way it would be. Mr. Torisawa indicated that there was simply no choice in the matter. If he were to return home, they would have to live separately. Also, Mrs. Torisawa stated that with her children growing they would need space to study, so they would need their own place. The parents agreed to this, but wanted to have supper and evening baths together. Bathing and eating are important contexts for generating intimacy within families and, thus, are often viewed as being central elements in building ties among and between family members (Clark 1994, Traphagan and Brown 2002). Mrs. Torisawa opposed this and they now live basically completely separate lives within the compound. Her opposition was based on an assumption, which she believes has been proved, that the gap between young and old is simply too extreme to allow for close living. Even within the compound, Mrs. Torisawa stated that the proximity has created a variety of problems and a great deal of stress for her, notwithstanding the advantages provided by being nearby, such as ready child-care:

> The way of thinking is totally opposite between the older generation and our generation. I don't have too much trouble with my mother-in-law and grandfather-in-law now because they have calmed down since we moved in [the grandfather-in-law is ill, thus she has very limited interaction with him]. Grandpa used to be the same as my father-in-law, but after he retired he relaxed or became more mild and better at interpersonal relations. But I really hate [*daikirai*] my father-in-law. There have been so many things that have infuriated me about his behavior. For example, I received a planter as a gift from some of our friends. My father-in-law thinks that our living space is under his control, so he will come and do whatever he wants to do around our house. What he did was, when I was away, he came and he saw the planter and thought it was useless, so he burned it as garbage. I was very angry and thought it was wrong for him to do that. So I told my husband that I wanted him to apologize, and also that I want him to buy the same thing to replace it because it was a gift. If our friends come to visit we want to have it here. So my husband told that to his father, but we never got anything—no apology, nothing. I don't re-

ally think that an apology would do anything, in any case, but I can't forgive him unless he does these two things for us.

We used to have a cow and one day he put a stick on the ground to chain the cow right outside of my kitchen window. I said, "I don't want this right outside of my kitchen," but he didn't listen. Either he didn't think that was a problem for us or he knew it was a problem and did it intentionally—I wasn't sure. I am never sure if he is simply insensitive or he is aggressively trying to cause problems for me.

Another time, we were collecting cans to put in a machine from which you get coupons to buy books. I wanted to do this as an incentive for my kids to buy books and it would be fun for them. My father-in-law came and just took the cans and threw them away. I told him why we were collecting the cans, but he did it again after that.

Mrs. Torisawa explained that from her perspective her father-in-law controls their lives. He feels that he is "number one" and has the power and right to control everything that goes on in the compound, including what happens inside the confines of the younger Torisawa's nuclear household. As she continued to talk, she indicated that her father-in-law lacks a sense that her nuclear family has a life independent of his, nor does he perceive any value in having fun as a family or having time to rest. She said, "He has been working all his life and doesn't rest—he always works. And he feels that we should be doing the same. If he sees us inside the house, he thinks we are lazy. So if there is some work around the [main] house or rice paddies, he will bang on the window and tell my husband to come out to help him." Mrs. Torisawa was so troubled by this pattern that she took a part time job, three hours a day, simply to get away from the household and her father-in-law. She said that the money was unimportant, she simply needed to have time away from her father-in-law.

To some extent showing the ambivalence in her feelings about her own nuclear family's relationship to her in-laws, she commented that after they moved there she had tried hard not to speak ill of her in-laws around her children and allowed her children to go to the grandparents house freely. However, the children no longer do so because they do not want to spend time with their grandfather. As is evident earlier in the chapter, Torisawa rather animatedly places the blame for the problem on the fact that the younger and older generations have completely different values (*kachikan*).

From Torisawa's perspective, differences in values make it impossible for the two generations to adjust to or accommodate each other. She shifts responsibility away from any particular individual and moves it to the circumstances of history that have shaped the two generations—pre- and post-war. The value sets embodied by the elder generation, as a result of being educated and socialized in the pre-war milieu, have created in that generation a different attitude towards concepts such as work, privacy, and family. To put this into more analytic terms, for Torisawa it is as though two distinct *habiti* exist in the different generations and, as a result, they are unable to fully communicate or deal with each other.

Understanding notions about the juxtaposition of *habiti* is fundamental to exploring the experience of aging in contemporary rural Japan. As Bourdieu argues, *habitus* refers to principles and structures which "generate and organize practices and representations that can be objectively adapted to their outcomes without presupposing a conscious aiming at ends..." (Bourdieu 1990:53). In other words, *habitus* refers to largely unquestioned structures that are embodied through mimetic transfer from the people one observes and with whom one interacts, as well as more obvious processes of socialization through education, discipline, punishment, and rewards. While Bourdieu is careful to avoid a deterministic conceptualization of the formation of *habitus* within an individual by recognizing the ability of people to improvise upon the basic structures of culture, the cognitive memory or cultural knowledge that one embodies throughout life limits the capacity of individuals to diverge dramatically from expected forms of performance. Indeed, we are inclined to reproduce basic performances, as it is essential to achieve cultural competence if we are to function in society and avoid stigmatization.

In the Japanese context, older and younger generations are largely viewed as having embodied distinctly different *habiti*. Their cognitive memory was developed from separate periods—pre and post-war— during which education (both formal and informal) was organized around different assumptions about the ways in which individuals should interact, particularly in terms of hierarchy within the family. The war experience itself, its subsequent deprivation, and the period of intense focus on building the economy that developed in the early post-war era are also closely linked to the *habitus* of the elder generations, having generated perceptions about waste and work that are viewed as distinct from younger generations. Indeed, it is really within this difference in *habiti* that the generation gap lies—a combination of particular historical circumstances and distinct approaches to education have generated a context in which there is a divide between young and old.

Understanding how younger and older Japanese think about their life situations, as well as the conceptualization of generational difference and its relationship to notions about cultural change, is important for understanding subjective concepts of well-being in contemporary Japan. Feelings of isolation and alienation and intergenerational conflict certainly have an impact on how people conceptualize their own lives and the manner in which they experience illness. Illness, of course, is also not simply a matter of the objective state of the health of bodies, but a matter of how people interpret their bodies in terms of notions of health, illness, and well-being. In the next chapter, we will turn more directly to a discussion of illness and aging and consider how Japanese conceptualize both cognitive and physical decline in later life and what this means for notions of health and illness among the elderly.

Chapter 3

Aging, Well-Being, and Ikigai

[H]ealth is not a universal fact, but is a constituted social reality, constructed through the medium of the body using the raw materials of social meaning and symbol.

—(Saltonstall 1993:12)

In the previous chapter, I explored some of the issues of alienation and isolation that have been associated with social change as it has affected the family and been exacerbated by the general aging of the Japanese population. Of course, with an increasingly aged population there also comes an increase in the number of people who experience chronic disease and, ultimately, who require long-term care. Some of the social services that have been developed to address this issue were discussed earlier; here I want to look at how Japanese conceptualizations of illness, health, and well-being are expressed in relation to the aging body. What identifies a person as sick or healthy? What are the causes of illness and health and how are conditions of health maintained? Answers to these questions, as is suggested by the quotation from Saltonstall above, cannot be limited to the causal, biological realm associated with biomedicine; instead one must also view the cultural context in which health and illness are experienced and interpreted. In the Japanese context, being a healthy older person is closely associated with being a good "old person"—a good *rōjin* (Traphagan forthcoming b).

As we move through this chapter, I will be developing the argument that health and well-being can be understood as a form of capital in the Japanese context. In one sense health and well-being are accumulated, embodied symbolic resources that people can tap into and by which they are judged on the basis of differential possession and the capacity to express that possession publicly. Health and well-being form an embodied state of capital that, in Japan, is closely linked to both individuals and groups and represents individual and collective abilities. Embodied capital can be generated and accumulated through investment in self improvement by enacting pedagogies of the body that are aimed at structuring bodies to fit within idealized conceptualizations of health and well-being. In other words, embodied capital, in the form of health and well-being, provides credentials and qualifications that certify individuals and groups as culturally competent.

In this chapter, I will use several theoretical terms that need conceptual unpacking. Specifically, the ideas of embodiment, capital, and power, which have been widely discussed in social science literature, require careful consideration. I will begin with the idea of embodiment. At its most basic level, embodiment is a form of memory. Memory, of course, is itself a complex concept that often eludes clear definition. Connerton provides a useful analytic framework for understanding memory. He views memory as consisting of three types: personal memory, cognitive memory, and habit memory (Connerton 1989:22). Personal memory is the set of rememberings that form one's personal history—the recollections of specific events that are combined to form a flow of time that represents the experiences of a particular person. This should not be viewed as the objective events that one has experienced over a lifetime, but as the remembrances of the events one has experienced, remembrances that are open to interpretation, reflection, manipulation, and representation. Furthermore, these remembrances do not exist in a void. Rather, they are continually constructed and reconstructed in concert with the other individuals with whom one traverses the life course—what Plath (1980) refers to as one's convoy of consociates—and who help in the process of interpretation and often even ascribe particular interpretations on events that are used in building those memories.

Cognitive memory involves the notion of remembering as a form of maintaining and recollecting meanings without any necessary connection to specific events or episodes in one's life. For example, as you read these words, you are engaged in a process of cognitive memory by which you are remembering particular words, concepts, and ideas, as well as the grammar and syntax necessary to string them together into coherent sentences. As Connerton notes, this type of memory does not require that the object of recollection be a thing of the past. Instead, it involves recollecting something that one has learned (embodied) or experienced *in* the past (Connerton 1989:22). This past experience is accessed and used in the present to interpret and make sense of present experiences.

Those of us who have had the experience of learning to ride a bicycle as a child, and then returning to ride again after several years' hiatus, have experienced the third form of memory—habit memory—in a very keen way. This is a form of memory that seems to be beyond the act of recollecting, instead being more of an autonomous motor reaction. As one gets on a bicycle and begins to ride, there is no conscious act of recollecting how to balance the bicycle—one simply does it. It can be argued (Bergson 1990 [1962]) that recollection and habit are distinct activities. The memory of how to do things such as riding a bicycle can be viewed a matter of motor behavior rather than memory per se and, thus, is very different from recollecting an event one has experienced or an idea one has learned. This points out the difficulties in trying to categorize different forms of memory. Breathing is also a motor behavior, but one that seems qualitatively different from riding a bicycle because it is not something we conceptualize as having been learned.

Drawing distinctions between different forms of recollecting has heuristic value in that such distinctions help us to think about different ways in which we remember, but dividing up memory into segments like this ultimately seems rather arbitrary. The differentiation between cognitive memory and habit memory is problematic if we think about the bicycle example. Clearly, one learns to ride a bicycle and the memory of how to ride a bicycle becomes a habit. Each time I get on, I do not think to myself, "how do I do this?" However, a long hiatus in riding may, indeed, invoke a brief period of uncertainty—the wobbly start—that requires a conscious recollection of memories about how to ride. My point here is that the concept of habit memory tends to treat this form of memory as permanent and beyond the scope of recollection—the durable structures, in Bourdieu's terms, that are embodied at a level so deep that we are unaware of the cognitive processes that come together in the act of recollection (Bourdieu 1977). Elsewhere I have argued (Traphagan 2000a) that the durable nature of these habit memories is open to question. Just as one embodies memories, one can disembody or unlearn those memories—even those perceived to be at a basic level of human being. This is true not only of cognitive memory via forgetting meanings of words or names of people, it is also true of habit memory. As is evident from the manner in which senility is conceptualized in the Japanese context, a person can unlearn *habitus* or habit memory. He or she can lose control of, or "forget", the basic assumptions about behavior that define one as human—in the Japanese case recognition of the interdependent and reciprocal nature of human interaction. In the process, one can also lose the symbolic and social capital that is associated with being a normal, culturally competent, human being. In the Japanese context, senility and other forms of functional decline in old age are closely associated with the unlearning of habit memory or of cultural competence.

This brings us back to the concept of embodiment, which I view as the combination and interaction of memory in the personal, cognitive, and habit forms. Our bodies, by which I mean the physical, mental, and social combination that forms a human, are in one sense themselves collections of past events, ideas, and experiences that are recollected and reinterpreted in the present. Through the performance of particular cultural practices—stylized movements and behaviors—we represent publicly a past that is "sedimented in the body" (Connerton 1989:72). This sedimented past is itself a representation, perhaps an artifact, of an individual's intersection with the cultural milieu in which he or she lives. But this sedimented past can also be disturbed when conditions of the individual body change. And this is where the second concept, power, comes into play.

Influenced by the work of Foucault (1978), Bourdieu (1977), and Gramsci (1971), the notion of power has come to be understood in terms of the interplay of resistance and domination that is interdependent and intersubjectively constructed as individuals and groups manipulate and interpret hegemonic and other forms that exist in society (Constable 1997:11). Foucault argues that rather than being static, power is brought together with knowledge through discourse, which he sees as neither stable nor uniform, but as "a multiplicity of discursive elements that can come into play in various strategies" (Foucault 1978:100). Discourse itself can be both an instrument of power and the result of actions by dominating forces that are exercising power; but it can also be a road-block or point of resistance that generates strategies opposed to the strategies of dominance used by elites (Foucault 1978:101). Foucault points out the ambiguities involved with discursive practice—that multiple and even contradictory discourses can occupy the same conceptual space and be strategically employed by the same people or institutions (Foucalut 1978:102). For Foucault, power permeates human relationships as it is exercised from innumerable social positions and is implicit in class relationships, knowledge relationships, sexual relationships, and so on. Even while power is exercised to dominate, there is no situation in which power is used without resistance or the potential for resistance being implied in the exercise of power (Foucault 1978:94–95).

Although Foucault's (1978:95) notion that power and resistance are found together appears accurate in many instances, in the Japanese case, particularly in relation to the elderly, the object towards which the use of power is directed and used—that object being the maintenance of physical and mental well-being through social interaction—is valued not only by those who are in positions of dominance, the government officials who invest their time and sometimes even risk political careers in the development of facilities intended for the maintenance of elder health, but also by the elderly themselves. As a result, although resistance sometimes can be found, for the most part, there is a fair degree of resonance between the interests of those in positions of power and those who might be viewed as being influenced by leaders who hold the political power necessary to develop programs for elders (Traphagan forthcoming a and b). Indeed, elders themselves, particularly men, are often primary players in the political power structure of towns like Kanegasaki and Mizusawa, as noted in Chapter 1 (Traphagan 2000c). Indeed, at the neighborhood level political organization can to some extent be characterized as gerontocratic (Traphagan 2000c). This should not be interpreted as meaning that the interests of the elderly and political leaders are always in tune. There are differences and conflicts; however, there is a general tendency for the interests of government officials and the general elder population to be similar not only because they both have a vested interest in maintaining the health and well-being of the elderly, but also because many of the political leaders are themselves elders.

Power, as it relates to the discourse on health and well-being in old age in Japan, is conceptually structured in terms of the concept of *ikigai*, which translates loosely as one's *raison d'être*, but which is better understood as a moral ideal that emphasizes self-actualization and self-discipline. *Ikigai* is employed by government officials as a means of encouraging older people to focus their primary attention on maintaining physical and mental health. While this is certainly beneficial to the elderly themselves, its use can also be understood as a subtle form of coercion in which old bodies are directed to become (self) disciplined bodies through the exploitation of the moral force contained in the concept of *ikigai*. I will return to a discussion of *ikigai* later in this chapter.

An understanding of how power operates is central to understanding embodiment; for memory is linked to the production of knowledge and control over knowledge is central in the development of hegemonic discourses that regulate the styles of practice that we embody (cf. Baer 2001). Well-being and illness are not only states of the body, they are also embodied states of knowledge and power that are often used to index the possession of cultural capital—the degree to which one is perceived as "fitting in" with ideals of selfhood and normative behavior.

Illness, Health, and Old Age in Japan

In her detailed examination of East Asian medical practices in urban Japan, Margaret Lock (1980: 218) notes that within East Asian medical practices (*kanpō*) Japanese orient the healing process around the sick person not as an isolated, diseased individual and his or her physician, but as being "at the center of an involved family." Sickness is not viewed as something experienced and responded to by an isolated individual, but, instead, is understood as a life course event in which one's immediate family, at least, share responsibility in relation to the healing process. In other words, there is a strong sense in which the healing process is conceptualized in terms of collective participation among the members of one's family. Lock employs Turner's (1977) conceptualization of liminality, a period of transition between social statuses or removal from normal frames of social interaction, to represent the experience of sickness not only for the individual, but for the family as a whole. The period of treatment is a time in which a person and his or her family are able, at least to some extent, to separate themselves from the normal responsibilities of society, such as work, so that they may focus their attention on returning the individual family member to health.

Although by no means unique to Japanese ideas about illness (see Hornum 1995), the concept of liminality takes on a particularly interesting dimension when the individual in Japan is terminally ill or has begun a process of cognitive decline associated with old age. The concept of liminality as Turner (1977), and before him Van Gennep (1960), use it, is based on the idea of a process of transition from one social status to another. The individual is removed from his or her initial status, marginalized in some way from the social whole (the liminal period), and then returned to the social whole in a different status. Terminal illness for Japanese is largely seen as a form of terminal liminality. However, instead of being placed between two different social statuses, the individual is in a situation betwixt and between life and death.

For the elderly Japanese, this liminal state is closely associated with two conditions that are central to understanding Japanese conceptualizations of health and illness in old age: *boke,* which can be roughly translated as senility, and *netakiri,* which means bed-ridden but implies considerably more than the state of one's physical body. Although the concept of senility in Japan overlaps with the North American understanding of cognitive decline in old age, there are several ways in which senility in Japan is conceptualized quite differently from the North American version. For the most part, Japanese recognize three categories of senility: Alzheimer's disease (*arutsuhaimā*), other forms of dementia associated with old age (*rōjinsei chihō*) such as vascular dementia, and *boke,* a term that defies direct translation into English, but connotes "being out of it" or a combination of physical and mental disorientation (Traphagan 2000a:135, 2002).

Arutsuhaimā and *rōjinsei chihō* can generally be understood as biomedical or clinical categories of disease. These conditions index pathological causes largely beyond the capacity of individuals to control. It is common for older people, in particular, to express their feelings about the onset of these conditions through the phrase "*shikata ga nai.*" This phrase is heard in numerous different circumstances in Japan, ranging from being late because a train was delayed to the serious realities of terminal illness. *Shikata ga nai* can be understood as a shrug of the shoulders indicating that "there's nothing one can do," but more is often implied. In a detailed discussion of the manner in which this phrase is conceptualized, Susan O. Long (1999:19) argues that stating *shikata ga nai* indexes feelings that at one level circumstances are beyond one's ability to control. However, as Long points out, use of the phrase in relation to the onset of terminal conditions such as Alzheimer's disease (AD) also may index attempts to maintain personal control over the process of dying and the changes in self associated with functional decline. In many respects, terminal illness and death are not significantly differentiated in the Japanese context; conditions like AD and cancer are conceptualized in terms of a loss of control that leads to an existence which "is no longer thought of as a truly human life" (Long 1999:19). This is the sense in which terminal illness can be understood as a form of terminal liminality in which one is neither fully a human life, nor has one yet died. Alzheimer's disease or other biomedical categories of senility index an individual who is either beyond the point of being able to exert effort, or to respond successfully to the efforts of others, to change the circumstances of life caused by the onset of the disease or in a circumstance where, regardless of what effort one exerts, it will make no difference in the outcome.

In contrast to AD and other forms of biomedically conceptualized forms of senility, *boke* typically is viewed as a category of illness over which people have some degree of control. Both in terms of its onset and progression, the concept of *boke* is expressed and responded to through a narrative that elaborates a theory of selfhood in which individual selves, as Dorinne Kondo notes, are not separable from the social contexts in which they are constructed, manipulated, and maintained. Indeed, Japanese government offices set up specific contexts which function as venues through which individuals can engage in a culturally circumscribed pedagogy of self-building that is enacted predominately through social participation (Kondo 1990:77). From the perspective of the government, while self-building is important for all individuals, it is the elderly—those at risk of losing the ability to engage in self-building because they have greater potential, due to their age, to experience or allow a reduction in activity—who have a considerable responsibility to involve themselves in these kinds of activities. *Boke* symbolically represents the disintegration of an intersubjectively constructed self and the loss of the ability to enact the pedagogies of self-actualization, particularly through participation in social activities, that are crucial to creating and/or maintaining ideal selves (Traphagan 2002, forthcoming a and b).

Having set up this trio of concepts related to cognitive decline in old age, it is important to emphasize that meanings associated with the term *boke*, in particular, are ambiguous. From the perspective of symptoms associated with the condition, *boke* is largely indistinguishable from AD as it is represented in North American (and Japanese) biomedicine. In some writing on the subject, the term is defined as simply a lay term for AD or other forms of biomedically defined diseases. One author argues that *boke* is represented as a broad lay term concept that includes AD and vascular dementia (Gonda no date). However, the manner in which specific symptoms are organ-

ized reflect Japanese conceptualizations of the person as being intersubjectively constituted via interaction with others (Traphagan 2002).
Symptoms such as memory loss and confusion are associated with
boke, but the condition is also sometimes somatized in terms of symptoms such as incontinence, hand stiffening, or balance problems. An
inability or unwillingness to engage in social interaction is also typically associated with *boke*—the *boke* individual may be viewed as having an inability to take on social and familial roles and to become
over-dependent (Kikkawa 1995).

Throughout the popular literature on *boke* there is no consensus
on how to define the condition. However, most authors agree that
boke has the potential to be controlled if one remains active and that
this differentiates the condition from AD. The idea that *boke* has the
potential to be controlled through activity links the concept to the
idea that self-building and effort are fundamental to being a good
person and are particularly important for being a good *rōjin*. Indeed,
the idea that one may have at least some degree of control over the
onset and progression of *boke* implies both a degree of hope that one
can remain a viable social entity and the idea that one *should* focus
one's attention and effort on doing whatever one can to ensure that
this happens. This taps into a basic moral value in Japanese society
that being active and giving one's all are fundamental elements of the
good person, in contrast to idleness, which is seen as contrary to both
individual and public well-being (Lock 1993:230–231, Traphagan
2000a).

Indeed, involving oneself in activities aimed at preventing or delaying the onset of *boke* is viewed as a social responsibility and, thus,
carries moral implications. Central to the moral content of *boke* are
ideas of reciprocity and interdependence, both of which are closely
connected to the Japanese conceptualization of selfhood as intersub-
jectivly constructed through social interaction. As *boke* develops, a
person gradually becomes removed from the interdependent relationships that define a human self as a social and, thus, moral entity
(cf. Plath 1980:217). *Boke* signifies a degeneration of the natural in-
terdependencies that are seen by Japanese as structuring human
selves, and shifts the person into an unnatural condition of unidi-

rectional dependence that negates the potential of the *boke* sufferer to reciprocate others for the help he or she has received in terms not only of care, but of the give and take that forms a basic pattern in Japanese social interactions (see, for instance, Befu's work on gift giving 1968). While in Japan any form of disability can take on this character of the unnatural, *boke* is particularly problematic from a moral perspective because it is viewed as something over which people may have at least some degree of control (Traphagan 2000a).

Collective and Individual Responses to the Potential of *Boke*

Elsewhere, I have discussed in detail the institutional frame in which people collectively engage in activities associated with preventing or delaying the onset of *boke* (Traphagan 2000a). Much of the basis of the social and collective elements of these activities can be summed up by a slogan that appears on the cover of a brochure for Kanegasaki's Center for Life-Long Learning (*shōgai kyōiku sentā*) a localized version of the *kōminkan* or government funded community centers found throughout Japan. These centers are often presented publicly as contexts in which people can employ pedagogies of self-building strategically to maintain personal health and well-being. The slogan tells us that the Center is:

> For the purpose of residents to carry on an abundant and bright life, an institution where one can be healthy through study, learning, sports, and recreation.

These centers typically consist of an office and several large rooms that provide space in which local residents gather for activities such as lessons on the tea ceremony, music, exercise, calligraphy, or, for the elderly, the Elder College (*kōreisha daigaku*) which organizes many of these types of activities specifically for residents over the age of sixty-five.

The *kōminkan* in Kanegasaki is more than simply a public facility in which people pursue hobbies and cultural activities. It is also a focal point where government officials and local citizens interact and a context in which government officials disseminate official rhetoric defining what constitutes a healthy community and healthy people, the two being closely connected. Numerous public documents are disseminated that indicate specific ways in which people can maintain healthy selves and, by extension of the individual into the social sphere, a healthy community. In general, these documents revolve around improving education and improving or nourishing one's self through involvement in hobbies and other activities aimed at self-cultivation. In one such document, the town charter, which is read aloud at most official public gatherings, townspeople are encouraged to "defend morality," "lead a healthy and safe life with cheerful mind and body," and make the town into an "hygienic" (*eisei*) environment (Traphagan 1998b). Work and production are also encouraged, as are building strong families, encouraging harmonious interactions, and respecting the elderly, children, and other people who are deemed in need of protection. The charter concludes by emphasizing the importance of public morality and devoting oneself to the improvement of society.

In many such government promulgated documents, health is defined not only in terms of individual well-being, but as an attribute of the collective expression of the individuals who coalesce to form a healthy community. A healthy community is built by focusing individual activity on self-actualization, which in turn recursively actualizes a healthy community. This idea implies not a neutral collective of individuals but a *moral* community in which individuals direct their personal activities in such a way as to generate communal well-being. This is accomplished through self-actualization, which forms the central means of building a good community and the fundamental pedagogy for creating disciplined selves and, through that, a disciplined community.

The concept of *ikigai* forms the basic theme around which activities associated with self-actualization are organized for the elderly.[1] The term varies considerably in relation to the specific practice to which it refers, but generally connotes one's purpose in life or something that one does deeply and wholeheartedly. There are few limitations on what can be counted as one's *ikigai*—*go*, beer drinking, flower arrangement, tea ceremony, *panchinko* (a form of arcade game), or gateball (team croquet, commonly played among the elderly) all might fit into this concept. The specific activity one chooses is highly personalized, although there is a tendency of people to group together for particular activities in terms of both age and sex. Elders tend to involve themselves in activities that are limited to only other people over the age of approximately sixty. And women throughout the lifecourse typically involve themselves in groups limited to their own sex, although this tendency is less pronounced with older women than it is with younger and middle aged women. While the choice of an *ikigai* is left to the individual, government bureaucrats may involve themselves in pointing older people in the direction of particular types of activities, such as cooking classes, which in addition to being presented as providing an *ikigai* are deemed important for ensuring good nutrition and are useful to widowers who may have had little or no experience with food preparation throughout their lives. Regardless of the activity, however, there is a basic assumption that having an *ikigai*, largely regardless of what it is, is a good thing. If the activity can be done in the context of a group of people who have similar interests, the potential of pursuing an *ikigai* for maintaining health and well-being in later life is greatly enhanced.

The relationship between the individual and group in the pursuit of *ikigai* has been discussed in detail by Gordon Mathews (1996:17, see also Traphagan forthcoming a and b). Here I want to emphasize that although having a particular *ikigai* is a matter of individual decision and is based on personal interests, the pursuit of the particular activity often implies commitment to a group of people with similar interests. Thus, the pursuit of an *ikigai* tacitly indexes one's involvement in socially oriented activities. This should not be construed as meaning the individual is in some way devalued or de-emphasized in relation to the group. Having an *ikigai* also indexes an introspective concentration of the individual focused on personal cultivation and growth. Indeed, it is personal growth that is often conceptualized as being at the root of community development and improvement. Thus, the social and individual aspects of *ikigai* are understood as being complementary in that as individuals reflexively engage in self-actualization, the communal whole reflects the positively oriented activities of the individuals within. In this framework, collectivities and individuals are not placed into a dualistic or oppositional relationship; instead, individually oriented activity is seen as inherently benefiting the group to which one belongs.

For the elderly, finding an *ikigai* around which to articulate one's identity often forms a central moral value, one that is advocated widely as a means of avoiding a lonely and illness-ridden old age. The moral content of this concept lies in Japanese ideas that often equate activity with moral behavior. As Margaret Lock (1993) argues, the individual who is lazy or idle is regarded as lacking in moral character. Central to Japanese ideals of the moral self are notions of doing. One who is active, particularly in the pursuit of self-cultivation, is following a path of good and moral behavior. By contrast, one who is lazy and idle is following a path that leads to personal decay and potential marginalization from society (for an interesting discussion of marginality and identity among day laborers see Gill 2001). For the elderly, having an *ikigai* is widely viewed as being the central method through which one may be able to avoid the onset of *boke*, although it is by no means seen as a guarantee. Nonetheless, as Mathews (1996:15) notes, an elderly person may feel sufficiently pressured, often through both the importance placed on this within the social milieu and from particular family members, to have an *ikigai* that he or she may actually be brought to consider suicide as a response to a perceived failure to focus attention on the pursuit of an *ikigai*. Recalling chapter 2, elder suicide has become a major social issue in rural Japan; several older informants interpreted this phenomenon in terms of *ikigai*, particularly when thinking about suicide among elders living alone. As one woman stated, "For those who are living alone, they become tired, they do not have any *ikigai*, and they are very pitiful [*kawaisō*] and they decide to commit suicide" (see Traphagan forthcoming a and b).

The rhetoric of *ikigai* is promulgated by the government through a variety of pamphlets, fliers, and other publications that are produced by local and prefectural government offices, and also by the association of Old Persons Clubs and other organizations that are focused on improving health and well-being among the elderly. Such publications emphasize the importance of having an *ikigai* and often depict elders engaged in hobby activities along with slogans such as *"ikigai* is the source of vigor", which appeared on the top of one government pamphlet on how to maintain health in later life.[2] In one publication by the Old Persons Club in Akita Prefecture that reports on an "elder college" held in the prefecture, several participants offered their post "graduation" comments on the importance of the "college" and of focusing one's attention in later life on having activities. Each of the participants began his or her comments with an enthusiastic title, three examples of which are below:

Let's all together make healthy inner selves [*kokoro*] and bodies

Let's respond that the Old Persons Club is the hope of society

Aim at the development of regional study activities

One woman described the school as bringing light to her inner self (*kokoro*), and most of the participants placed the importance of the school in their own lives within the broader context of building a sound community. As is evident from the second quotation above, some even presented the Old Persons Club as the vanguard of hope for the future of Japanese society. While this may be an overly ambitious goal, this particular quotation and many others paraphrase or borrow from the rhetoric promulgated by local and prefectural government offices, which place socially oriented activity in the broader context of community improvement and which emphasize the role of the elderly in leading these efforts. In this particular publication, it is indicated that one of the central elements in the elder college was the idea of promoting senior sports leaders to encourage older people to engage in physical activities that help in maintaining health. Again, this carries the broader consequence of improving the entire community.

The emphasis on finding an *ikigai* in later life forms one key element in the rhetoric of self-articulation which I have been discussing and which focuses on the idea that constructing disciplined selves through the pursuit of an *ikigai* will not only generate individual health and well-being, but also will generate communal well-being (Kondo 1990:107). Older individuals (indeed, this applies to people of any age, but is particularly important for the elderly) who orient the articulation of self toward the pursuit of an *ikigai* engage themselves in a kind of transformative power that is used to maintain not only personal well-being, but the well-being of the community as a whole. This form can be understood in the sense that Foucault suggests in his discussion of the idea of discipline, as "a technique for the transformation of arrangements" (1977:146). I do not intend to imply that other aspects of having an *ikigai* are unimportant; people may pursue a particular activity for the pleasure or interest. However, it is also the case that the discipline associated with having an *ikigai* organizes individual bodies and the cognitive expressions of those bodies into networks of (power) relations that structure activity in terms of idealized forms of the good or model person. One can imagine here the model patient, the A-student, or the well-behaved child. The concept of (self) discipline encapsulates the practice of aligning one's own behavior closely with patterns of behavior associated with an ideal or idealized person. For the elderly, this means that to be active and to be engaged in pursuit of an *ikigai* is to be a good *rōjin* (Traphagan forthcoming b).

The alignment of self-articulation within the scope of idealized forms of behavior has practical consequences in that the more closely one is aligned with the ideal, the more able one is to accumulate cultural capital through the recognition that one is engaging in disciplined behavior. A self-disciplined individual is engaged in the act of self-cultivation, which can be seen as an inner-directed form of transformative power aimed at cultivation of personal health and well-being, and this has social consequences. Through the pursuit of an *ikigai*, older individuals discipline themselves by orienting the articulation of self around activities associated with the *ikigai* ideal. Disciplined selves individually represent a disciplined community and the well-being of these individual selves indexes a community that, itself, is disciplined, (morally) healthy, and doing well.

Power, Well-Being, and *Ikigai*

As I have noted elsewhere (Traphagan forthcoming b), if we think about the personal health consequences of pursuing an *ikigai*, a Lévi-

Straussian structuralist approach comes to mind in which *ikigai* and functional decline in later life are set in a binary opposition that also indexes the opposition between positive and negative forms of behavior (Lévi-Strauss 1974). In some respects, this approach accurately represents the relationship between illness and *ikigai*—a central element in maintaining good health is being active physically, mentally, and socially and one of the best ways to do this is through pursuit of *ikigai*. By contrast, inactivity and illness are closely linked together. Idleness, particularly when it is manifested in the form of an unwillingness to engage in socially-oriented activities, is seen as a precursor to decline in individual well-being. In comparison to other members of society, the elderly are perceived as being at greater risk of this potential because slowing down is viewed as a normal part of the aging process.

Through the above consideration of concepts of health, well-being, and illness, it becomes evident that for Japanese there is a close relationship between the individual and the social in terms of how health and illness are conceptualized. While Japanese fully recognize the identification of illness with infectious diseases or other forms of pathology such as cancer and genetic predispositions for problems such as diabetes, the historical background of the relationship between health and illness also has involved a close linkage between the potential for burdening others with illness and social ostracism of the sick person. In the past, as Lock points out, the sick person "became a burden to his or her family; illness was associated with rejection from society, and as such it was greatly feared" (Lock 1980:25). Illness was associated with pollution, and as a result required ritual treatment in the form of baths and various herbal medicines that generated a physical reaction in the body that could be interpreted as having expelled polluting agents (Lock 1980:25). This concern over cleansing the body continues to be important in contemporary Japan; although not necessarily interpreted in terms of pollution, one can routinely find agents that are ingested with the idea that they will clean out the body. Often these include some form of alcohol combined with another element that increases its purifying power. Examples include *mamushi shōchū*, a form of clear alcohol made with potatoes in which is placed a poisonous snake (*mamushi*), the venom from which is said to envigorate and cleanse the body. Another example is saké (known as *kinpaku-iri*) in which gold flakes have been added, which also is said to cleanse the body.

While the close relationship between illness and pollution lacks the weight it once had in Japan, the social connotations of individual illness continue to be important aspects of Japanese medical conceptualizations. Lock (1980:226) argues that for the sick, the responsibility for dealing with health and healing lies within the family, rather than the individual specifically. This conceptualization of responsibility for health and healing is multi-directional. While responsibility for health lies with the family, the individual also has a responsibility *to* the family to do everything he or she can to maintain his or her personal health and well-being. Indeed, within the government rhetoric that surrounds *ikigai*, this responsibility is extended beyond the confines of the family to apply to the community as a whole.

It is important to recognize that the responsibility which lies at the center of this is less one of actually avoiding sickness than it is one of making a genuine and sincere effort to avoid sickness. Blacker points out that in relation to specific acts that can lead to uncleanliness from the perspective of the Shintō deities (*kami*)—such as menstruation, birth, disease, snakebite, or bestiality—pollution and polluting acts typically lack any moral content, instead being viewed as "unavoidable concomitants of the human life cycle" (Blacker 1975:42). Indeed, illness, too, is seen as an unavoidable part of human life, and functional decline in old age, including the onset of *boke*, is largely viewed as a normal part of the aging process. But the fact that these conditions may be viewed as normal, and in some ways even expected, does not mean that one lacks responsibilities in relation to their potential onset.

Indeed, the concept of *ikigai* indexes a conceptualization of well-being that emphasizes the morally framed idea that by pursuing an *ikigai* one is practically and symbolically making a sincere effort to maintain physical and mental health, thus, reducing the potential of burdening one's family and one's community. This concept is closely tied to the idea of *gambaru*, which is a central moral element in the pedagogy through which people construct disciplined selves (see Singleton 1993). For older Japanese, more important than simply having an *ikigai* as a means of maintaining health and well-being in old age is the idea that, regardless of the actual outcome, one should be constantly making every effort possible to maintain health—and the pursuit of *ikigai* is viewed as the best way to do this, indeed in some ways the pursuit itself is synonymous with effort. If one is pursuing an *ikigai,* one is inherently engaged in effort directed at maintaining health and well-being, and through that, doing whatever one can to avoid burdening one's family and one's community with provision of care.

It is via personal effort that transformative power is exercised individually in relation to the attempt to control health and well-being in old age. Through the use of power in this sense, individual older people are able to embody cultural capital that is associated with being a good *rōjin.* The pursuit of an *ikigai* is a practice aimed in large part at avoiding the onset of *boke,* but the consequences of that onset are more than simply a matter of potentially staving off cognitive decline. To become a "*boke rōjin*" or to fall into another category of decline such as "*netakiri rōjin*" or bedridden old person, is to risk the implication that one did not make sufficient efforts to avoid that state (see Long 2003). The state of being *boke,* in particular, forms a type of social death in which an individual is no longer able to engage in the social interactions that are basic to defining one as a person. In other words, the pursuit of an *ikigai* is a tactic in which power is employed to maintain physical, mental, and moral health. It is the combination of these two aspects of the person that form the basis for understanding well-being in the Japanese context.

For Japanese, being active, particularly when it involves situating oneself in social settings, is seen as inherently good. This is unrelated to age—anyone who pursues activities aimed at self-improvement is seen positively and is viewed as doing something that is a natural part of being a healthy, well-adjusted human (Lock 1993, Traphagan 2000a). For the elderly, however, the pursuit of an *ikigai* has specific implications related to the fact that functional decline, and for men an abundance of free time, are perceived as a normal and expected part of the late life course. The elderly are perceived as being at greater

risk of sliding into an inactive life and, ultimately, a life of dependence upon others for care. Pursuit of an *ikigai* is a use of power focused inward; it is power aimed at what Long describes as "directive
control" intended to manipulate changes in self (physical and mental) associated with the aging process by manipulating the "most basic
sense of who one is" (Long 1999:23).

But the strategic use of the concept of *ikigai*, and concern over
maintaining health in old age, is by no means limited to individual
activity. Government officials routinely place activity for older people into the framework of *ikigai*, encouraging the elderly to build
selves that accord with ideals associated with the good *rōjin*. This underscores the fact that in Japan having a healthy mind and body is
more than a matter of personal concern—it is a social responsibility,
one particularly important for the elderly to recognize given that they
are at increased risk of functional decline in comparison to other age
groups.[3] Government officials strategically deploy the concept of *ikigai*, and the centrality of self-actualization through having an *ikigai*,
as a moral frame through which the elderly can express—through
doing—their own willingness to contribute to the social whole by
being good *rōjin*. This should not be interpreted as meaning that old
bodies in Japan are simply subject to forces of dominance over which
they lack control. Instead, the doing of *ikigai* generates cultural capital in the form of adhering to ideals about how a good self is articulated (Traphagan 2000a:174).

As I have shown throughout this chapter, cultural capital associated with being a good *rōjin* is structured around the notion that
healthy individuals form a healthy community. Indeed, health and
well-being themselves can be understood as a form of capital that indexes a person who is, by virtue of being healthy, making efforts to
adhere to the ideal of the good *rōjin*. In many respects, this capital is
closely related to the idea that concern with oneself and one's own
health and well-being index a broader concern with the community
in which one lives. In this sense, there is no sharp distinction between
inner directed concern and outer directed concern. Concern directed
toward the self is inherently also directed toward the community in
which one lives, because it is individuals who make up that commu-

nity. I do not want to suggest, as has so often been done, that Japanese people are groupist and that this is an example of sublimating the individual to the group. Quite to the contrary, the idea that concern about one's inner health and well-being affects and indicates broader concern is related to the idea that it is through interaction with others that individuals are most fully expressed and realized. This idea does not devalue the individual, but places the well-being of that individual into context, overtly recognizing that individuals are not isolated entities but are intertwined with other individuals through social relationships. And, indeed, the well-being of the group is itself dependent upon health and well-being of the individuals of whom it is comprised.

What is most interesting for my purposes here as I move into the following chapters is that these social relationships are not limited to the mundane, living world. The context of social interaction in which well-being and concern are enacted includes ancestors, spiritual entities (*kami*), and humans, all of whom are interconnected, at least in part, via ritual performance. In the following two chapters I will turn to the manner in which older people use religious ritual as one way of expressing individual and collective concern and consider how this is related to ideas of health and well-being.

Chapter 4

Omairi: *The Practice of Concern*

She placed on the altar the traditional seasonal offerings for Bon—things that the soul of her brother might like: eggplant, green grapes, cucumbers, tomatoes, sake.

Sake? For her brother? "Even if he died of too much sake," she told me quite seriously, "on this special occasion he should enjoy it."

—(from Bumiller 1995:105)

Ritual behavior associated with shrine visitation and ancestor veneration in Japan is organized around what I will present in the next three chapters as a total life care system[1] that is used to enact worldly benefits and well-being for oneself and one's family, one's community, and one's nation (cf. Reader and Tanabe 1998) and through which people enact concern. This life care system involves various sets of reciprocal relationships, such as those between *kami*[2] and humans or living and dead, which are enacted to ensure and maintain personal and collective well-being. Rituals associated with ancestor veneration are particularly important elements in this reciprocal and interdependent life care system. In terms of reciprocity, the *kami*, ancestors, and living are linked through social interactions enacted in the context of ritual performance. This is particularly pronounced in relation to ancestor veneration. On the one hand, the living keep the ancestors socially involved in the living world through ritual ac-

79

tion and provide for them through food offerings, while at the same time the ancestors are seen as watching over and protecting the people whom they have left behind. As one Buddhist priest put it, "There is a feeling of give and take between the living and the dead. The ancestors protect the living in return for the giving of offerings of rice."

Although exchange is normally a central feature of this relationship, this is not necessarily balanced, and providing for the well-being of the ancestors is more complex than the mere provision of food and other offerings. In much the same way as one's children and other family members need love[3] and attention, ancestors also need to be loved, cared for, and thought about. The manner in which one expresses attention and emotions directed toward one's ancestors is largely through ritual performance. Ancestor veneration rituals serve to keep the dead attached to the world of the living through a combination of affective and material bonds. The ritual obligations associated with reciprocal care are the basis for an interdependent and complementary relationship between living and dead. There are also practical consequences of ensuring that the dead are remembered through ritual performance; without ritual attention, there is a risk that the ancestors will become *muenbotoke*, which literally means 'unattached spirits' (Smith 1974).

The point I want to emphasize here is that both roles—that of the living and that of the ancestor—are structured around ideas of supplication and nurturance (*amaeru* and *amayakasu*) that are more broadly evident in the structure of Japanese social interactions. Japanese psychiatrist Takeo Doi has written extensively on the structure and content of this relationship as it is conceptualized among Japanese. He argues (1973:99) that *amae* represents a form of dependence in which people seek "identification of subject and object," rather than simply an attempt to depend upon another person. This form of dependence assumes an intersubjective relationship between individuals in which both supplication and nurturance are exchanged and there is an assumption of some degree of mutual identification between those involved. Too rigid a distinction between the *amae* and *amayakasu* roles should be avoided. Indeed, in the case of the relationship between ancestors and descendents, it is clear that both take on the nurturing role simultaneously, and ancestors and living not only reciprocate, but also depend upon each other for nurturance and care (cf. Lebra 1976:240).

Existing simultaneously in both roles, nurturance and supplication are central to the co-construction of the relationship as the living and the ancestors depend upon each other for their continued well-being and, ultimately, for their existence—the living would not exist without the ancestors, and the ancestors depend upon the living to keep them involved, as memories, in the world of the living and to provide the basic love and attention that all humans require. In other words, living and dead are mutually involved in enacting and maintaining each other's well-being. At the center of Japanese ritual activity is concern; both in the immediate sense of concern with the well-being of friends and family, both dead and alive, and in the sense of Tillich's notion of ultimate concern. For Japanese these two forms of concern are merged—ultimate concern is expressed in terms of immediate concern with the well-being of those with whom one interacts on a daily basis, with one's community, and in some cases even with the entire nation.[4]

In this chapter, I will consider some of the main aspects of personal ritual participation in Japanese society. I suggest that, for Japanese, rather than being organized around doctrine or institutional affiliation, religious activity is centered on the idea of concern about personal and collective well-being. Ancestor veneration is one element in a basic disposition towards pragmatism in religious behavior among Japanese, who emphasize action in the form of ritual performance and de-emphasize doctrinally grounded systems of belief and exclusive commitment based upon beliefs in specific deities or doctrines (Musick et al. 2000; Reader 1990:16). As they engage religiously related forms and structures, Japanese people use a blend of institutionally connected symbols and ideas in often idiosyncratic ways depending upon particular needs at particular times (Smyers 1997). A lack of strict institutional orientation to religious activities is one reason that, for Japanese, it is not unusual for a person to engage in Buddhist, Shintō, and even Christian forms of worship and ritual under different circumstances without experiencing conceptual or affiliational conflicts (Mullins 1998:141).[5]

More important than the institutional frame in which a practice is located, Japanese concern themselves with situation and the instrumental aims associated with a particular form of ritual activity. That is, Japanese are concerned with observing ritual actions that are appropriate for a particular need. For example, one goes to a Shintō shrine or in some cases a Buddhist temple to pray for success in high school entrance examinations, the recovery of a loved-one from sickness, returned affections by the object of one's desire, and so on. In recent years, some Buddhist temples have become frequently used locales at which to relieve feelings of guilt or distress following an abortion through participation in a ritual known as *mizuko kuyō* (Hardacre 1997; LaFleur 1992:4). Specific shrines and temples are often known for and in many cases market themselves as being particularly useful in requesting specific benefits, such as scholastic achievement or a sudden death in old age, devoid of prolonged and incapacitating illness (Traphagan 1998a; Wöss 1993).

Historically, institutional lines themselves have been hazy. Much of the present-day institutional separation of Shintō and Buddhism can be traced to 19th Century political aims directed toward developing an indigenous state religion. This served to emphasize Shintō over Buddhism, which arrived from continental East Asia in the 7th Century (Hardacre 1989; Kitagawa 1966:201), although during the Edo Period (1600–1868) population was tracked through the association of families with Buddhist temples, a practice of institution building which led to the formation of temple parishes (*danka*) which I discuss below. During the Meiji Period (1868–1912), while the separation of politics and religion was formally enacted into law, nativist ideologues, powerful in the Meiji government, engaged in anti-Buddhist and pro-Shintō activities aimed at erasing "ancient evil customs" via the "removal of all Buddhist priests, acolytes, and retainers from Shintō shrines throughout the nation" (Ketelaar 1990:9). Indeed, the Meiji period witnessed persecution of Buddhism such that it has been estimated that over 40,000 temples were closed or destroyed, thousands of priests were laicized, and numerous temple artifacts were ruined (Ketelaar 1990:7). The persecution Buddhism experienced in the early Meiji period faded as Buddhism began to reposition itself and find new ways to express its relevance in the context of a changed and changing Japan (Ketelaar 1990:214). Indeed, by the 1920's the Nichiren sect of Buddhism was influential in its expressions of patriotism and antidemocratic, anticommunist sentiment; as Herbert Bix notes, many of the upper-echelon military officers and right-wing civilian ideologues were members of the Nichiren sect (Bix 2000:164).

It is not within the scope of this volume to explore the historical aspects of the separation of Shintō and Buddhism, rather my point is that the post-Meiji Restoration separation of institutional Shintō and Buddhism was something imposed by political authorities rather than inherent in the ways people historically have practiced the two religions. Even with this imposition in the 19th Century, as Smyers points out in her superb study of the Japanese deity known as Inari, Japanese people did not embrace this division and a lack of partitioning of Japanese religious behavior on the basis of institutional forms continues to be common into the present. For example, she notes that in some places Inari is worshiped as a Buddhist deity, in others as a Shintō deity, and one informant indicated that it "may even be the same as the Christian God" (Smyers 1999:7). In one of the neighborhoods in Kanegasaki, there is a religious monument dedicated to a Buddhist deity known as Fudō (who is invoked for protection from disasters such as fire), although it is constructed in the form of a Shintō shrine. Each spring the head priest from the largest Shintō shrine in Kanegasaki comes to perform a purification ritual, with the members of those families connected to this smaller religious monument in attendance. The issue of whether or not the religious site is Buddhist or Shintō is irrelevant to those who attend, and when asked participants have difficulty identifying it as one or the other. They simply refer to the shrine as Fudō-sama (honorable Fudō) and continue the ritual activities that have been conducted at the shrine for generations, without concern for the institutional basis of those rituals.[6]

Sectarian Affiliation

The limited importance of exclusivity in terms of major sectarian membership is readily evident by looking at how Japanese report religious affiliation. The Japanese Agency for Cultural Affairs holds an annual survey of religion that tracks sectarian affiliation, numbers of clergy, and numbers of places of worship (see, for example, Bunka-chō 1995). Figure 4.1 shows religious adherents by sect, total adherents, and the total population of Japan in five-year intervals from 1975 to 2000. By looking at the columns for total religious adherents and the Japanese population, it is immediately evident that Japanese people indicate multiple membership in religious sects—total affiliation is close to double the population of the country. This is predominately due to the fact that most Japanese will list both Shintō and Buddhism as religions to which they have an affiliation, which raises a question of the extent to which the institutional division between the two religions is meaningful in the minds of Japanese. Members of less mainstream sects, such as the quasi-Buddhist Sōka Gakkai or Christianity, are unlikely to list membership in more than one sect because these sects tend towards exclusivism from a doctrinal perspective. But the vast majority of Japanese represent themselves in surveys as being both Shintō and Buddhist, or perhaps a better interpretation is that they represent themselves as not being one or the other—the institutional orientation of affiliation is not particularly relevant.

To be sure, it would be difficult for Japanese to list themselves in any other way. While distinctions are often made between Shintō and Buddhism—for example purity rituals and weddings typically are associated with Shintō, while funerals and veneration of the dead are associated with Buddhism (cf. Norbeck 1954:119–120)—participation in specific rituals is much more directly linked to calendrical cycles and life course events than with sectarian differentiations. Membership in a particular shrine or temple is usually connected to one's membership in family and community. In the case of Buddhism, people do not usually belong to a particular sect of Buddhism on the basis of belief, but, rather, on the basis of a combination of geography and historical family affiliation. Temples have parishes that are often connected to the neighborhood in which they are located, and families that constitute the parish keep the family grave site at the temple, which automatically generates an affiliation with the sect of that temple.

Figure 4.1 Sectarian Affiliation and Total Population for Japan 1975–2000 (in thousands)

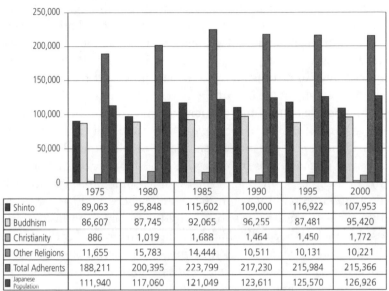

	1975	1980	1985	1990	1995	2000
■ Shinto	89,063	95,848	115,602	109,000	116,922	107,953
▢ Buddhism	86,607	87,745	92,065	96,255	87,481	95,420
▨ Christianity	886	1,019	1,688	1,464	1,450	1,772
■ Other Religions	11,655	15,783	14,444	10,511	10,131	10,221
■ Total Adherents	188,211	200,395	223,799	217,230	215,984	215,366
■ Japanese Population	111,940	117,060	121,049	123,611	125,570	126,926

Source: Japan Ministry of Public Management, Home Affairs, Posts, and Telecommunications
(http://www.stat.go.jp/english/data/nenkan/zuhyou/b2117a00.xls)

This is not to suggest that membership in a particular Buddhist sect is invariably tied to geography or proximity—it is not unusual for a family or an entire neighborhood to be linked to a temple some distance away or for different families in the same neighborhood to be linked to various temples. There are instances in which commitment to a particular faith/sect is the basis of belonging (Andreasen 1998), but geography, in terms of proximity to one's family grave and the temple associated with it (if there is one), and kinship play a central role in defining the limits of parish membership. In order to understand the close connections among kinship, place, and sectarian affiliation, it will be helpful to explore the case of one hamlet in Akita Prefecture.

Yamada[7] is a hamlet of twelve households located in a picturesque valley nestled between dark green mountains to the north and south. The valley is very narrow—no more than three quarters of a kilometer across at the wider parts and the houses sit up against the southern mountain at its base and overlook the rice paddies to the north. There is a single winding road that runs through the middle of the hamlet and two small roads off to the north, both of which go up into the mountains. The roads, wide enough for only a single car to pass at a time, are paved within the area of the houses but quickly turn to dirt just beyond the last house. At the west end of the hamlet, and at the end of the paved segment of road, there is a large pine tree on top of an artificial mound around which are three tiered rings of stone. On the top of the mound there is a gravestone and at the base of the mound an altar area where people can burn incense. This mound is the collective grave for the deceased of all of the households in the hamlet, as well as some houses connected through kinship linkages but located elsewhere, and has served in that capacity for at least two-hundred years, and continues to be used in the present. Both officials in the town government and local residents noted several times that this was one of the few remaining collective hamlet graves in Japan, thus it should not be taken as representative of burial practices throughout Japan. However, the burial of affinal and consanguineal kin in a common grave is the normal form of burial in Japan.

Kinship links among the households in Yamada are closely related to sectarian affiliation, thus it is important to go into some detail about these links. Japanese kinship patterns are organized around the stem-family system (known in Japanese as the *ie*) in which different households are linked together through a main household (*honke*) from which branch families (*bunke* or *bekke*) can form.[8] The main household and its branches are tied together through genealogical links to a founding ancestor, patriarch of a line of eldest male heirs (at least ideally, although it is often not the case that the eldest males are always the successors) who hold the position of head of household. Each branch forms its own segment, with its own head of household and branches that can themselves form new branches.

Figure 4.2 is a map of the households in Yamada and shows the links among the households in the hamlet. Indeed, all of the households in the hamlet are linked together through a connection to

Figure 4.2 Yamada hamlet in Akita Prefecture

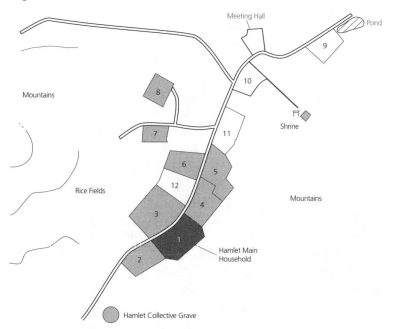

household number one, which is the main household for the hamlet. All of the households in the hamlet go by the family name of Nara and all are either directly or indirectly connected to the main household. The households shaded in gray are branches of household number one—which is the *honke* to the entire hamlet. Those that are white, are branches from branch families, known as *magobunke* or grandchild branch. Thus, the households that are direct branches from number one, are 2, 3, 4, 5, 6, 7, and 8. Household number 3 has itself had two branches (9 and 12) in its history. Number 8 also has a branch (10), which itself at one time had a branch that no longer exists in the hamlet, having moved to Osaka so that the family could live near the son's wife's relatives when the grandmother in that household died. This family is not expected to ever return and is no longer considered to be part of the hamlet, although some hamlet residents were uncertain about its status because there had never been a clear declaration of separation from the hamlet. The house in which the family lived has been demolished and the land it occupied is used by one of the residents of the hamlet for his business of carpentry. Finally, number 11 is a branch from number 5. The number of branches from household number 1 are considerably greater than those in Yamada. There is another hamlet not far away from Yamada that has an additional twelve households that are branches from the main household in Yamada and according to the wife of the main household, there are a total of 40 branches, with greater and lesser degrees of social connection to the main household.

This system of kinship relations is important for our discussion here because it is closely related to several aspects of the religious life of the community. All of the households are tied together by the fact that they use a common grave. Indeed, when I used the word *"hanareta"* which means "to have separated" to describe the relationship between the *honke* and *bunke* in the hamlet, the wife of the main household (number 1) was uncomfortable with the term, indicating that because all of the families continue to use the same grave, they are not truly separated. Were there to be a separation in which a branch family did not use the grave in Yamada, I was told, it would be more common to use the term *bekke* rather than *bunke*. This distinction bears similarity to data obtained by Keith Brown (personal communication) concerning the meanings of these two terms as identifying kin and non-kin links between branch and stem families. *Bunke*, according to Brown, can be understood as a branch household in which kin links exist, such as in the formation of a branch household for a sibling of the heir such as a brother or sister; *bekke* represents the creation of a branch via a non-kin link, such as setting up a branch household for a former tenant or servant who has given many years of dedicated work to the main household. In the case of Yamada, the kinship linkage among the *bunke* to the common ancestor of the hamlet is closely maintained through ritual performances.

While all of the households in Yamada have Buddhist altars (*butsudan*) located in them, the main household for the hamlet has the largest. This *butsudan* occupies a separate building attached to the main house, a magnificent traditional style Japanese building comprised entirely of *tatami* rooms and covered by an enormous tile roof. The house is surrounded by exquisite gardens with sculpted maples and pines that can be viewed from the *tatami* rooms in which the family entertains guests. On a hot day, the doors slide open to the garden and across the house to make a pleasant breeze. This house forms a *de facto* temple for the hamlet, as none of the residents belong to a temple close to the hamlet. The temple for the hamlet is located in Akita, about twenty kilometers away. According to the elder wife in the main household, their large *butsudan* was erected so that the hamlet members could carry out ritual performances there—it was too difficult to go back to Akita to conduct the rituals that needed to be done on a regular basis. The head of the main household functions as the leader for rituals that take place in the main house, thus he might be viewed as a lay religious leader although he stated that he has no formal training.

All of the households in the hamlet belong to the Pure Land sect of Buddhism (*jōdo shinshū*), but they do not belong to the same parish (*danka*). Three of the households, 3, 12, and 9 belong to a temple in another part of the town in which Yamada is located. It should be immediately evident that these three households are related in that both 12 and 11 are branches of 3. This kinship link is central to understanding the parish affiliation of these households. During the Meiji period (1863–1912), household 3 resigned its membership in the temple in Akita City and shifted to the one closer to Yamada, taking 12 and 11 with it. This was not done for practical reasons of distance, but for reasons of kinship. This shift occurred when a daughter of household 3 was married into a temple family for the temple known as Shōkokuji. According to the wife of the main household, "they went to the other parish because the wife was moving into that temple as a priest's wife and moving the three households over would strengthen the parish and make it easier for these households to conduct temple-related worship. Because she went from the main household of the group, the entire group went as well."

The importance of kinship in religious practice in Yamada is also evident in the rituals that are carried out in the hamlet. Most important among these are the ancestral veneration done on the 28th of each month, the festival of the dead (*obon*), and the vernal and autumnal equinoxes (*ohigan*). Monthly ancestral rituals are held on a rotating basis throughout the hamlet; the ritual is held at a different house each month moving from one house to the one next door, although there is no set pattern or rotation according to residents. The one exception to this rotation is on the 28th of November. This date falls in the period known as *oshimotsuki*, which in Yamada is celebrated from the 21st to the 28th and in other areas from the 23rd to the 28th of November, commemorating the death of Shinran, the founder of the Pure Land sect. The ceremony conducted on the 28th primarily focuses on the idea of returning *on* or gratitude to Shinran, but also is practiced as a means of returning *on* to one's ancestors (*hotoke*) more generally.

The November 28th ceremony is always done at the main household, as are ceremonies connected to the collective grave at the festival of the dead in August (*obon*) and the vernal and autumnal equinoxes (*ohigan*). The monthly ceremonies are attended by those households in the immediate hamlet; representatives of other households linked to the main household do not participate. On the 7th of August, however, representatives from all of the households with individuals buried in the collective grave visit in order to clean the grave and the area around it. There is also a ceremony held at the main house in which representatives from each household gather to pray at the large *butsudan*. These ceremonies are not attended by all members of the households, but, instead, are attended by one or two representatives from each household, who are normally members of the elder generation in that household.

From these examples, we can see that membership in a particular parish is not necessarily a matter of geography; it may also be a matter of practical considerations related to kinship ties. The marriage of a daughter into a temple household led to the shifting of one branch and its associated branches to a different parish in order to strengthen that parish. Indeed, it is difficult to separate the ritual activities performed in the hamlet from kinship ties. Decisions about who leads and which household carries out which responsibilities are closely related to relative positions of households within the overall family system. At the center of this is the main house, which has the responsibilities for leading ritual performances and for maintaining the main altar for the entire stem-family.

In the example of Yamada, we can see some of the complexities of parish and sectarian affiliation that accompany religious participation in Japan. Affiliation is not necessarily, or even primarily, organized around commitment to a particular "faith." Instead, people belong for reasons of family history, proximity to a particular temple, or associations among and between families that have social consequences not necessarily directly connected to religious matters. In other words, sectarian affiliation is not generally oriented around theological questions. This point extends beyond the realm of sectarian affiliation to the realm of the manner in which Japanese enact ritual and ceremonial performances.

Omairi: Ritual Expression of Concern

The primary way in which individuals engage in religious ritual in Japan is through the practice of *omairi*—visiting or "prayer" which can take place at the family grave site, at a temple or shrine, or at the various ritual sites inside and outside of one's home. *Omairi* is a term that can be translated as prayer (another word for which is *ogamu*), although the content of meaning does not entirely overlap with conceptualizations of prayer as they are understood in non-Japanese religions, thus I will refrain from using the English term here. *Omairi* can be associated either with Buddhism or Shintō and involves a complex of meanings. The *kanji* (Chinese character) used for the term literally means to participate or take part in something. In its verb form, the character indicates the performance of an action, but can also imply a return to one's origin (as in *mairimasu*).[9] It is in this sense (of a return to one's origin) that the concept of *omairi* has particular salience for Japanese in reference to ancestor veneration. To do *omairi* at one's family altar (*butsudan*) or grave site (*ohaka*) is to return to one's origins in the form of visiting with one's ancestors—the peo-

Figure 4.3 Stone shrine known as *myōjin-sama* protects
a residence in Jōnai

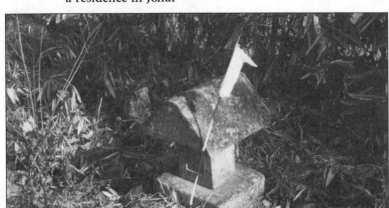

ple who have gone before and given life to those who are currently alive.

The importance of this practice rests in the fact that *omairi* is the central activity employed in maintaining individual and collective well-being via ritual performance. As noted above, there are two basic locales at which one does *omairi*—in the privacy of one's home and at public sacred spaces such as temples and shrines. In terms of ritual performance, *omairi* can involve a range of activities that vary somewhat from person to person and from household to household. There are also regional differences in the types of locales and specifics of ritual practice that occur. For example, in Kane-gasaki people often have a small, stone shrine placed near their house, often at the northwest corner of the property, which is known as *myōjin-sama* (see Figure 4.3). At this monument, offerings are made to the "outside deity" that protects the household.

Common throughout the area that was formerly the Date feudal domain (*han*) during the Tokugawa era, these monuments are not found a few kilometers to the north, which was in the Nambu domain. Another example of this kind of variation can be found in the fact that in Iwate Prefecture and many other parts of Japan, the *kamidana* (deity shelf, discussed below, see Figure 4.4) is not usually placed in the same room as the *butsudan*, however in neighboring Akita Prefecture it is common to find the *kamidana* placed directly over the *butsudan*.

Not only do the specific places at which *omairi* vary somewhat from one region to another, it is normal for households in the same area to exhibit variation in the particular sacred spaces that are used as well as in the particulars of rituals performed at those spaces. For example, some households will have a *kamidana* while others will not. In Yamada, there are *kamidana* in some of the households, though not in the main house. While offerings are made to the Shintō deities at these sites, some of the residents indicated that this was relatively unimportant in comparison to Buddhist ritual practices and is also a recent development. As one man in his sixties recalled:

> During the war, the government wanted everyone to have a *kamidana* [god shelf] in their houses to protect the nation. In the houses where there is one, it is because they built a new addition for the *butsudan* and put one in at the same time. But the original houses in this area didn't have *kamidana*. It was a result of political decisions in the war aimed at protecting the nation. There were no *kamidana* in houses generally prior to that time.

In fact, when I queried the wife of the main house in Yamada about the statue of a fox associated with the deity Inari that was placed in the hall outside of the room with the *butsudan*, she explained that it had nothing to do with having Shintō religious objects in the house, per se, but that it was a gift and they did not have any other place to put it.

Patterns of ritual performance also vary in detail from one household to another, even while the basic forms of ritual observances are consistent, involving offerings of food and drink. For example, on a single day of going from house-to-house in Jōnai in Kanegasaki to map the positions of *myōjin* monuments, I found differences in placement, despite the fact that the local priest had told me that it should always be placed in the northwest corner of the property facing southeast, and I also found differences in the specifics of ritual offerings made to the deity at virtually every house I visited. Below are excerpts from my fieldnotes from that day:

- The *myōjin* here is obviously not cared-for...the homeowner and I walked out to the back of the house and the top had been knocked off. The resident of the house put it back on, but there was no evidence that they ever do any ritual practice there and he indicated that they do not use it. The shrine is placed at the south end of the property and faces north.
- At this house there is a *myōjin* set up in the northwest corner of the property against the wall facing southeast. I was told that the family was of samurai descent and that is why they have it. They give uncooked rice (*kome*) on the first of each month, but they do not give water or saké at this time. On New Year's Eve, they give uncooked rice, rice cakes (*omochi*) and rice with red beans used for auspicious occasions (*sekihan*).
- The *myōjin*, which the wife of the household called "*soto-kami-sama*" (outside deity) is placed at the east side of the property facing west and slightly south. She said that the orientation of the myōjin-sama is related to the house. The house faces east, rather than south, thus the myōjin-sama is placed to face inward toward the house.
- I talked to the wife in this household, who was out in the garden weeding. It obviously hurts her back a great deal because she was quite hunched over and could not stand up straight to talk to me, instead sitting down on the stoop and looking up at me. The *myōjin-sama* on her land faces south. They do rituals on the 1st and 15th of each month. On those days they give salt and water. Also, on the 9th, 19th, and 29th of September they give rice with red beans and do this at suijin-sama (the deity for the well) also. On New Year's Day, they

give two small pieces of rice cake (*omochi*). She said that the myōjin-sama was east-facing in the past and on the south border of the land. But a priest told them that it was not in a good position. The priest came and they burned the spot where it had been located after moving it to the new position. Then it was o.k. to use the old position for anything. After it was put in the new position, the priest conducted a ritual to purify the area.

- I met Mrs. Saito and we went to see the *myōjin-sama* which is placed at the back, southeast corner of her property. She said that they put it on a concrete cinder block because the land there was kind of low and they thought they should raise it, although no priest had indicated this was necessary. Also, the direction of this is facing northwest. She said that it is different from everybody else around here (and commented on my map as showing that) and they have wondered if they should move it to another position because they do not think it is a very good position. But they have not done anything about it.

Just as the presence of shrines in the household varies, attitudes about the importance of conducting rituals at Shintō religious spaces, such as the *kamidana*, vary considerably, even within the same family. For example, Nakamura Juro, who was in his forties when we talked, stated that the first thing his father does when he comes home with his pay envelope is to put it on the *kamidana* for a while and then retrieves it later. His parents also put an arrow for exorcising evil spirits (*hamaya*) that they purchase at the local shrine each year on New Year's Day on the *kamidana*, as well as other important objects such as gifts. Responding to his parents' behavior, Nakamura said that he has never gone to the *kamidana* and laughed at the idea. Although it is doubtful that he has, in fact, never done *omairi* at the *kamidana* in his house, even as a child, this illustrates the considerable variation even within a single family about the importance of, at least, Shintō objects, spaces, and ritual practice.

Figure 4.4 *(opposite page)* These photos show examples of *kamidana* in houses located in Kanegasaki. The upper photo is from a farmhouse and the lower one is from a merchant household. Note in the lower picture the *maneki neko* figurine to the right, often found in businesses or merchant (and other) households to bring wealth or financial success. The paper in the lower right shows a schedule of areas to be visited during the election for the town assembly. The main room in this house was being used as the election headquarters by a candidate for the assembly.

The Private Context of *Omairi*

Within the context of one's household, *omairi* is typically done at the Buddhist altar (*butsudan*), Shintō god shelf (*kamidana*) (see Figure 4.4), or at another sacred space such as myōjin or suijin monuments in one's yard. In general, *omairi* involves a combination of offerings, most often in the form of food, and contemplation of, or a request to, the deities or one's ancestors. As noted above, many of the households in the communities where I conducted fieldwork have *kamidana* either directly over the *butsudan* or in an adjacent room. The *kamidana* usually consists of a small shrine made of wood—that is basically a model of a large shrine building—in which is placed an amulet that either symbolically represents the deity protecting the household, or in many cases, is actually referred to as the deity itself. The *kamidana* is placed high up on a wall, usually about three-quarters of the way to the ceiling. There is a sacred straw festoon that has paper streamers hanging from it and which is hung across the front of the *kamidana*, symbolically marking the purity of the space. In some cases votive tablets, known as *ema*, on which messages to the deities are written are hung from the bottom of the *kamidana* and small stands on which offerings are made rest at the front. One can find various sacred objects, although not necessarily together, on the *kamidana*. One may find an arrow or other objects such as food offerings on or under the shelf.

The extent to which people involve themselves in *omairi* directed toward the *kamidana* varies considerably from one household to an-

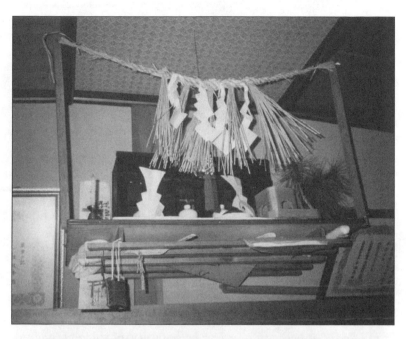

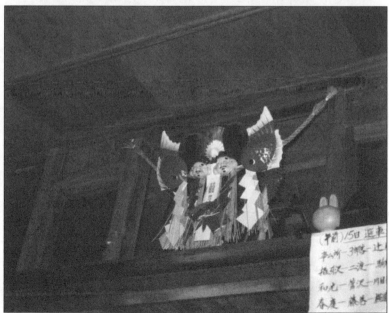

other. In one household, for example, the *kamidana* was above the *butsudan* and the grandmother indicated that she gives offerings of rice at the *kamidana* every morning at the same time she gives offerings to the ancestors at the *butsudan*. She also indicated that she always goes to the *butsudan* first, because the ancestors are more important than the *kami*. In this particular household, offerings are rarely made in the evening, either at the *kamidana* or at the *butsudan*—but in other households offerings are made in both the morning and at night, typically corresponding with the serving of breakfast and supper. Rice is commonly given to the *kami*, as is water or saké. I have also seen vegetables such as daikon offered at the *kamidana* during the New Year's holidays, as well as rice with red beans, which as noted above symbolize success or an auspicious beginning. Typically, when an offering is made, the person making the offering first lights votive candles kept on the *kamidana*, following which he or she claps his or her hands twice and holds them together for a moment with eyes shut, standing silently in front of the *kamidana*. An individual may ask the deities for something in particular, such as health for his or her family, or may have no specific thought in mind.

In some households, people do not regularly visit the *kamidana*. One man in his fifties explained this tendency by invoking the Japanese saying "turn to the *kami* in times of trouble" (*komatta toki no kamidanomi*), which indicates that people visit with the *kami*—either at the *kamidana* or at a shrine—only when a need arises. While offerings and requests to ensure individual and familial well-being are made at the *kamidana* by most people who have one at New Year's, the extent and style of *omairi* at other times of the year varies from one household to the next.

As noted above, the wide variation in the particulars of ritual performance done at the *kamidana* are also reproduced at other household Shintō-related objects such as *myōjin* and *suijin*, and variation is also evident in rituals performed at the family altar or *butsudan*. More than with *omairi* at the *kamidana*, variation in whether or not family members make offerings at a *butsudan* is closely related to the particular circumstances of a household in terms of whether or not a member has died. Indeed, if no immediate member of the household has died, it is unusual for a family to have a *butsudan* at all, although it is by no means prohibited.

> At my house, we have a *kamidana* and a *butsudan*. My father died December 6th. So every month on the sixth day a priest from my temple visits to chant. Before he comes, we have to prepare a dish with rice and other things [to give as offerings]. I don't do it, my mother prepares for that. The Buddhist priest will spend about ten minutes of chanting and he is supposed to get 2,000 yen for the work.

Like *omairi* at the *kamidana*, *omairi* at the *butsudan* varies considerably from one household to another. Unlike *omairi* at the *kamidana*, however, in additional to personal and household differences, there are also sectarian differences that reflect variations in approaches to ancestor veneration evident within the sects of Buddhism. In particular, members of the Pure Land sect of Buddhism may chant or think the phrase "*namu amida butsu*" which is an invocation of the name of Amida Nyorai, the Buddhist deity of infinite light. Sincere utterance of this name is said to lead to automatic admittance into the Pure Land or Buddhist heaven. The considerable microvariation in practices related to ancestor veneration and *kami* worship in Japan has been noted by others (Smith 1974, Smyers 1999), but it will be illustrative to present some of the variation in Jōnai and Yamada.

Although anyone can do *omairi* at any time in life, care of the *butsudan* (and the *kamidana*) is typically the work of the elder members or of the middle-aged housewife (*yome*) in a multigeneration household, or the housewife in the event that there is no elderly generation at home. The fact that women are more often responsible for doing *omairi* may be connected to their role in the family as taking care of domestic work such as cooking, since daily *omairi* usually involves making an offering of rice and water.

In general, *omairi* at the *butsudan* involves placing the offering on the altar, lighting candles and then incense from the candle flames, ringing a gong or striking a hollow wooden block, and placing one's hands together in front of one's face or on one's lap, closing one's

Figure 4.5 Woman having just completed *omairi* at
the *butsudan* in her house

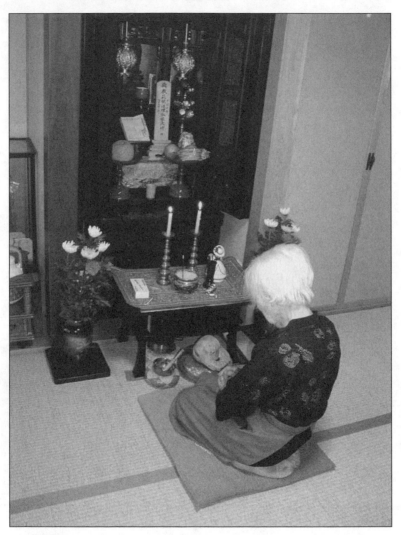

eyes, and spending a minute or less in this position. Figure 4.5 shows
a woman just after completing *omairi*—the candles have been lit and
incense is burning. In this case, the incense is placed into the ash pot

Figure 4.6 A smaller, apartment-sized *butsudan*

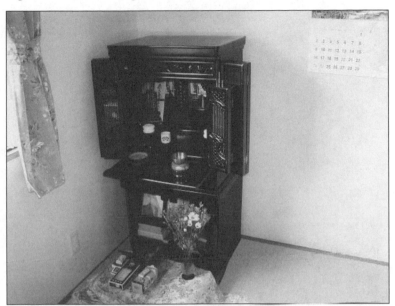

for burning the incense in an upright position. In other households, the incense may be placed on its side in the pot—it is customary to ask when doing *omairi* as a guest at someone's house how the household places the incense.

The *butsudan* can range considerably in size, from a small, apartment-sized altar such as that pictured in Figure 4.6, to an altar that takes up its own room. Figure 4.7 shows a *butsudan* of the larger variety that is typical of those found in houses in the Tōhoku area. It fits into a segment of the wall that is designed for the *butsudan* and is placed next to an alcove known as a *tokonoma* where art objects such as arranged flowers and a hanging scroll, that may be a religious text, are often placed. Some informants stated that in addition to daily *omairi* at the *kamidana* and *butsudan*, they also do *omairi* at the *tokonoma* indicating that this can be considered a sacred space in the house, although it is by no means always seen in this way. *Butsudans* vary in their contents, but they will consistently have an *ihai*, which

Figure 4.7 A larger *butsudan* typical of those found in a house

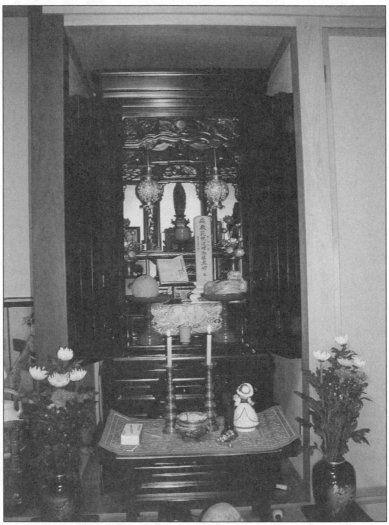

is a votive tablet on which is written the posthumous name (*kaimyō*)
of a deceased member of the family. There will be one *ihai* for each
family member who has died, thus a family with a long lineage may

have numerous *ihai* on the *butsudan* and may not have clear knowledge of the living identities of the individuals who are enshrined.

As noted earlier, offerings made at the *butsudan* may include many foods other than rice and water. Special foods, such as melons, that a family has received as a gift will be taken to the *butsudan* and placed there for the ancestors to enjoy.[10] Guests who visit a household in which they knew a family member who has died will often go directly to the *butsudan* in order to memorialize the deceased friend or relative. It is common for guests to bring a gift of something that was enjoyed by the deceased. For example, in one case of a man who died suddenly at the age of 68, those who visit his widow often bring ice cream because it was among his favorite foods. In one household, a few months after the funeral of the grandfather who was well-known in the area as a farmer, the family was still receiving regular guests who brought offerings to Grandpa. At one point, there were two cartons of cigarettes placed by a guest at the *butsudan* as an offering to Grandpa, who dearly loved his tobacco. This was in spite of the fact that no-one else in the household smoked. Eventually, the cigarettes were given to the brother of the head of the main household because he was a regular smoker. Indeed, most of what is offered to the ancestors at the *butsudan* is ultimately consumed by the living. Food and drink offerings are not wasted—even the very small amount of rice, less than a handfull, that is offered daily to the ancestors may be returned to the ricemaker to be rewarmed and consumed by the family later in the day.

During the period in which one remains quiet in front of the *butsudan*, most informants state that they think about their ancestors or make a specific request. One woman, who was 82 when we talked and belonged to the Jōdo Shinshū sect of Buddhism, said that when she does *omairi* she repeats "*namu amida butsu*" over in her head several times. She also asks for the well-being, health, and happiness of her family. In this woman's case, it is her parents who are memorialized on the *butsudan* and she lives in a three-generation household including her son and his wife and their children. Another woman, who was 84, said when I asked about *omairi*, "do you mean for the ancestors [*hotoke-sama*, a word that can refer to the ancestors or to Buddha] or Shintō deities [*kami-sama*]?" I asked if they are different and she replied that "for the *kami* you clap and for the *hotoke* you put your hands together." It is interesting that she did not go into detail about how the entities enshrined differ, but instead focused on how the actions one takes in relation to those entities differ. This woman gives rice every morning to the ancestors and asks both the ancestors and the *kami* to protect her living family.

A woman of 66 told me that she asks for the health, happiness, and success of her family from both the *kami* and ancestors, and a man of 83 explained that he previously did *omairi* every day at the *butsudan* and *kamidana* but stopped when he was around 80 because his physical condition made it difficult to move around. He said that he does *omairi* occasionally, and when he does, he thinks about his ancestors and asks them to protect his family. A 91 year-old man said that he asks the ancestors and *kami* to help his family avoid sickness and to do well. He believes that he does *omairi* for both himself and for his family and takes rice to the *butsudan* every morning and often claps in front of the *kamidana*.

These examples indicate the variation in the specifics of worship and also the fact that there is not a strong differentiation between what is done at the *kamidana* and what is done at the *butsudan*. However, most informants indicated that it is *omairi* at the *butsudan* that is most important in their lives and that it is necessary to consistently carry out this type of ritual performance, although, again showing the microvariation in practice and ideas related to ritual performance, one woman in her late eighties stated, "the *kami* are more important because they are a more general and, I think, powerful thing." These examples also point to a central theme in the practice of ancestor memorialization: death is not a time of separation from the household or family. Rather death is a time of transition where individuals take on a new role within the household upon death. Ancestors remain as vital members of the family, who are thought about and of whom requests are made. Hamabata (1990) gives a good example of this when he describes entering an informant's house and being taken directly to the *butsudan* to be introduced to the father of the family who had recently died. He also notes the general tendency to, for example, open the doors of the *butsudan* during special events occurring in the house so that the ancestors, who are in some ways seen as being located in the memorial tablets, (cf. Smith 1974) can partake of the proceedings.

The Ancestors

As can be clearly seen from the preceding paragraphs, the ancestors remain an important part of the household. But, who are the ancestors? Robert J. Smith (1974) and David Plath (1964) have both looked at the identities of the ancestors who are memorialized in the *ihai* on a family *butsudan*. Smith conducted a census of the people memorialized in which he found that it was not unusual for family members to be uncertain about the identity of some of the individuals memorialized. Plath (1964:301–303) has identified three broad categories of ancestors: the departed, the ancestors, and the outsiders.

The departed are those ancestors who have died in recent memory—those for whom there are still living members of the family who can remember them. This category may also include relatives not directly from the household, but who were close to members of the household who want to keep their memory alive. It is not unusual for memorial tablets of the departed to be copied, by a Buddhist priest, and included on more than one *butsudan*, such as the *butsudan* for the main household and a branch household. One of the women with whom I spoke lived in Akita City more than 500 kilometers from her natal home in the Tokyo area. She had purchased a small *butsudan* for her apartment (Figure 4.6), on which she had a memorial tablet for her mother, who was also memorialized on the *butsudan* in her natal home. She stated that she had a copy made in order to have her mother closer to her. The ancestors, in contrast to the departed, are those for whom there is no longer any clear memory of the person as an individual identity. These deceased form a broad collective of ancestors of the entire past of the household. Finally, outsiders are those who do not have direct connection to the household. For example, Smith (1974) notes an instance of finding a memorial tablet that represented an individual who had died near the house in which he was memorialized. While these tablets do not normally occupy the same status or location on the *butsudan* as family tablets, they are kept in order to prevent the deceased from becoming a wandering spirit and potentially bringing trouble into the household for lack of proper ritual attention.

The process through which the dead traverse the conceptual space from living to departed to ancestors is structured through ritual performance. Several authors (Beardsley, Hall, and Ward 1959:343, Smith 1974, Ooms 1967) have described a ritual process in which individuals are moved from the position of departed to that of ancestor via ritual performances that occur on the 7th, 49th, and 100th days after death, and then on the 1st, 3rd, 5th, 13th, 25th, and ultimately the 33rd or 50th anniversaries of the day of death. These rituals involve bringing family members together at the household altar, as well as at the family grave where the ashes of the deceased are collectively entombed beneath the gravestone, for rituals that are conducted by a Buddhist priest. Ooms argues that the lifecourse and deathcourse are punctuated by a set of rituals conducted as one moves through different transitional periods. Examples of these rituals include *omiyamairi*, when newborns are taken to a Shintō shrine either approximately one or three months following birth (this varies by region), and *shichi-go-san*, when girls of 3 and 7 and boys of 5 years of age are dressed up in elaborate kimono or other dress clothes and taken to the shrine for a brief ceremony and to have formal photographs taken. Other important points in life where one engages in ritual activity include *seijinshiki* when an individual is recognized as an adult at the age of twenty, marriage, *kanreki* at the age of sixty indicating entrance into old age, and the funeral and ancestral ceremonies described above. There are other points in the lifecourse where one may engage in ritual activities related to transitions, particularly those associated with *yakudoshi* or inauspicious years (which I will discuss in chapters 6 and 7).

Specific, personal experience of the departed is a central feature in determining how the deceased are conceptualized. Without a direct linkage to a specific ancestor who was known by the living, the ancestors are generally understood in terms of a collective mass of predecessors, who, although impersonal and ethereal, continue to be understood as being involved in the reciprocal rights and obligations that characterize interactions among the living (Plath 1964:303). In other words, they continue to be part of the social life of the household as "ancestors", but not as specific departed individuals whom the living continue to remember and memorialize through ritual practice. Both the departed and the more amorphous ancestors are implicated when people discuss ancestral protection of the family, but in many respects it is the departed who are most directly conceptualized as being actively involved in the protection of the living.

While the departed are particularly salient in the lives of the living, the power of the ancestors to influence the actions of the living should not be underestimated in Japanese society. It is important to understand that conceptualizations of what the ancestors actually are vary considerably from one person to another. Some people see them largely as an abstraction, rather than a specific group of spiritual entities. Others clearly see the ancestors as spiritual beings who, at least in terms of the recently departed, have defined identities. The same type of variation can be seen in understanding the location of the ancestors. When asked where the ancestors are located, informants indicated they are on the family altar, in the family grave, or simply everywhere in a very abstract sense.

Feelings of close relationships between the living and dead appear to become stronger when one has experienced the death of an intimate relative or friend. In detailing their own life histories associated with religious and ritual participation, several informants indicated that the emotional experience of doing *omairi* changed after the death of a loved one. As Oikawa Hiroko explained:

> When I was younger, I just went to the *butsudan*, put my hands together, and did *omairi*, but I didn't have any feeling about it. I had no mind [*shin*] when I did *omairi*. But now I have a very different feeling. Now when I do *omairi*, there is a deep feeling in my *kokoro* [center, heart, mind]. I feel the *omairi* much more. This change occurred when my mother-in-law died.

For Oikawa, the death of her mother-in-law gave rise to a more meaningful and visceral sense that the ancestors were watching and protecting her family. This can be understood in terms of Rappaport's notion of high-order meaning, in which there arises an awareness or conceptualization of unity or identification between things previously viewed in a more distinct way. In Oikawa's case the death of her mother-in-law led to a feeling of identity with the deceased akin to Rappport's notion of a "radical identification or unity of self with other" (Rappaport 1999:71), although the extent to which this can be viewed as "radical" in Rappaport's use of the idea is open to question. What is clear is that for Oikawa, regular experience of this identity or unity comes in the form of a direct link between the living and the dead that is maintained through the enactment of ancestor-related rituals, particularly those performed on a daily basis at the family altar.

Although people do not necessarily move through life constantly thinking about the desires of their ancestors, perceived desires on the part of the dead do come into play in decisions about behavior. The power of the dead to influence directly or indirectly the lives of the living is particularly evident in Hardacre's work on the ritual known as *mizuko kuyō* for aborted fetuses, stillborns, and children who die early in life. As Hardacre notes, perceptions among some Japanese about the potential for aborted fetuses to negatively affect the lives of women, in part as a result of their not having been appropriately cared for via rituals similar to those used in ancestor veneration, are an important motivation behind carrying out these rituals, as well as an incentive for religious entrepreneurs to prey on those fears and profit from conducting the rituals (Hardacre 1997, see also La Fleur 1992).

Mizuko kuyō is a particularly clear example of the concern among the living about the power of the dead, but other less dramatic examples exist as well (this example is also discussed in Traphagan 2003b:131). During the summer of 1996, one of my informants was hospitalized and then required to spend over a month in bed resting as a result of over-working himself while planting his rice fields during some unusually hot days in May. When I asked him why he continues to plant the rice, even at the risk of his health—and, indeed, his life, given that his problem was a heart condition—he responded that having received the land from his ancestors, he had an obligation to care for it (Traphagan 2000a:58–59). The implication of caring for the land was that it had to be farmed, rather than allowed to go fallow, because producing something from the land was an indication that it was being properly used and cared for. Another informant, who constantly complained about having to weed her property, explained that her family had received its land some 300 years ago from the feudal lord (*tono-sama*) of the hamlet in which she (and I) lived, thus she had an obligation to him and to her ancestors to keep the land neat and well maintained.

The Public Context of *Omairi*

In the preceding paragraphs, I have explored *omairi* largely as it is expressed and experienced within the confines of one's home. The private expression of *omairi* extends into more public spheres via specific, family-oriented forms of ancestor veneration that take place at grave sites and temples—particularly at the summer festival of the dead known as *obon* and at the vernal and autumnal equinoxes when people visit the family grave and clean the grave and areas around it—and are visible to others. I would argue, however, that these forms of veneration remain fundamentally private, for although they occur in public spaces, they are only engaged in with other members of one's immediate family. There are, however, contexts in which individuals participate in public, if not collective, forms of *omairi*. These forms of *omairi* are often intertwined with other kinds of activities, particularly with travel and sightseeing, as visitation at shrines and temples is a popular form of tourism in Japan.

In the remainder of this chapter, I want to focus on the practice of *omairi* as I have observed it at the temple complex located in the town of Hiraizumi, in the Kitakami river basin, a few kilometers south of Mizusawa and Kanegasaki. The site is famous throughout Japan for its historical importance as the seat of the northern Fujiwara military family that held political control over the region in the twelfth century and maintained about 70 years of sovereign power over the northeast area of Honshū with administrative, economic, and political independence from the capital of Japan in Kyoto (Fujishima 1961, Yieng-pruksawan 1998). During its period of power, the Fujiwara family amassed a huge fortune from locally produced gold, part of which was used to build replicas of the temples and shrines of Kyoto, as well as a palace, a replica of which has been built in the town of Esashi, just north of Hiraizumi, that was used as a set for an NHK drama on the Fujiwara and is now a tourist attraction. The town has long been re-membered as a site of important military battles—the poet Bashō vis-ited there in 1689 and reflected upon "the dreams of soldiers past" (in Yiengpruksawan 1998:1). The plains visible from the temple comlex are said to be the site of the great warrior Yoshitsune's (1159–1189) last stand, where he had been driven by his enemies along with his mighty vassal Benkei (see Totman 1981:85–91).

In 1105 the initial lord of the family, Fujiwara Kiyohira, restored the temple known as Chūson-ji, which was originally established by Jiaku Daishi in 850 AD and Fujiwara Motohira, Kiyohara's son, es-tablished the temple Mōtsū-ji in the middle of the twelfth century. Hiraizumi became the center of the "gold culture" (*ōgon bunka*), that flourished in the 11th and 12th Centuries and is said to have rivaled the sophistication and extravagance of Kyōto. Chūson-ji, on which I focus here, is situated on a small mountain on which there are nu-merous temple halls that one can visit and at which one can do *omairi*. The original, twelfth century, buildings at Chūson-ji were largely destroyed when the fourth lord of the Fujiwara, Yasuhira, was defeated by Minamoto Yoritomo in 1189 (Fujishima 1961, Yieng-pruksawan 1998:4). All that remains of the original site are the sutra depository and the Konjiki-dō, a stunning temple hall extravagantly covered in lacquer and gold leaf that is kept inside a special building where one can view the hall after purchasing a ticket for ¥1,000. The original structures at Mōtsū-ji were destroyed by fire in 1226, and like Chūson-ji the structures have been rebuilt, mostly since the seven-teenth century. Today both temples are prosperous.

Chūson-ji has since 1958 been the seat of the Tendai order of Bud-dhism for the Tōhoku region and, as Yiengpruksawan (1998:4) notes, today there is a constant stream of pilgrims and tourists who come to do *omairi* or to view the extensive collection of Buddhist artworks and architecture on the grounds of the temple mountain and experience its natural beauty. At the base of the mountain, there are numerous restaurants, some serving *wanko soba,* a form of all-you-can eat noodles that are popular in the Tōhoku region as a tourist draw, and souvenir shops that sell a vast array of religious objects such as Buddhist prayer beads (*juzu*) and scrolls, as well as toys, postcards, key chains, and lacquered objects such as soup bowls and chopsticks. The competition among these restaurants and shops is considerable, and middle-aged women often stand in front of the stores saying "*irasshaimase*", inviting customers to come in and spend their money.

At the center of the souvenir shop area, there is a large parking lot where one can pay to leave one's car while visiting the temple, and across busy Route 4, the main north-south route through this part of Tōhoku, there are more restaurants and large parking areas for the busses that continually arrive with school groups on field trips and tour groups on holiday. The two temples at Hiraizumi, Chūson-ji and Mōtsū-ji, are among the most popular tourist attractions in the Tōhoku region and draw visitors from throughout Japan. However, the fact that it is a tourist draw should not be viewed as diminishing the religious significance of the site, nor the importance of doing *omairi* as part of the practice of visiting the temple complex. Indeed, the two are not easily distinguished, as Smyers (1997, 1999) has pointed out in her work on the deity known as Inari mentioned above.

As one walks up the long, steep hill, with tall and ancient cedar trees along the sides, it is difficult not to be impressed by the beauty and history of the temple complex. The forest to the right and left of the main gravel path is a lush green; the ground around the trees covered in a carpet of moss. At various points along the path there are stone lanterns and other objects, on which pilgrims have placed hundreds of smooth pebbles, as is customary at many sacred sites in Japan. The exact purpose of placing these stones is not clear to most of the people with whom I have spoken although all were aware that this is something done as people conduct pilgrimages to sacred locations. One woman who worked at one of the booths selling religious objects along the path did place this into a more theological context when she indicated, with a note of uncertainty, "I think they are for going to heaven [*gokuraku*] and are placed when ascending a sacred hill and are a matter of faith (*shinkōteki ni*)." About half-way up the hill, there is a small noodle restaurant and immediately next to it the first temple hall where one can do *omairi*. Off to the right there is a path that diverges from the main path and takes the visitor through a long series of bright red *torii*, arches that are typically placed at the entrance to a Shintō shrine. This path represents an alternate entrance to the temple complex and there is a small shrine devoted to the deity Inari as the path enters into the woods.

Continuing to walk up the hill, the first major building one comes to is Benkei-dō (also called Akodo-dō). For several years of visiting Hiraizumi as a tourist, I had thought that this was in fact a Shintō shrine (*jinja*) because there is a large *torii* at its entrance. During a conversation with a woman who sells *omamori*, or protective amulets, at a stall next to Benkei-dō, I learned that it is in fact a Buddhist temple (*otera*) and that the *torii* was simply a remnant of an earlier shrine that had been located on the same spot that had been destroyed, again reminding one of the lack of concern about sectarian divisions that characterizes much of Japanese religious practice.

Benkei-dō is one of several temple halls along the route to the main temple, each of which is viewed as being powerful for coping with specific (health) problems or for ensuring general health and well-being. By doing *omairi* as one visits the different temple halls, one engages the deities and can protect oneself from misfortune by so doing. At the booths in front of each temple hall, one can purchase *omamori*, or small silk, metal, or plastic amulets and talismans that are considered by some to contain the powers of the deities enshrined at the sites where the *omamori* are purchased (Reader 1991:23) and that are used to protect one from misfortune (see Figure 4.8). *Omamori* are widely purchased in Japan to protect against misfortune such as traffic accidents (people hang the *omamori* in their cars), illness, or to help in achieiving a particular goal. The meaning of the term *omamori*, which derives from the term *mamoru* (to protect) as it relates to protection from either Buddhist or Shintō deities is not uniform, nor is it often discussed or specifically thought about. For example, when asked how ancestors (*gosenzo*) and *kami* protect peo-

Figure 4.8 Both of the *omamori* pictured indicate that they are for the purpose of blocking the onset of *boke*. The one on the left indicates that it is specifically for the purpose of helping those who are normally healthy to "accomplish" the containment or prevention of *boke*. The term *nasu* is used and means to accomplish as it is written on the card, but the same sound also can mean eggplant (with a different *kanji* character). Thus, this *omamori* is made in the form of an eggplant. The *omamori* on the left was purchased at a Shintô shrine and the one on the right at the Chûson-ji temple complex at Hiraizumi.

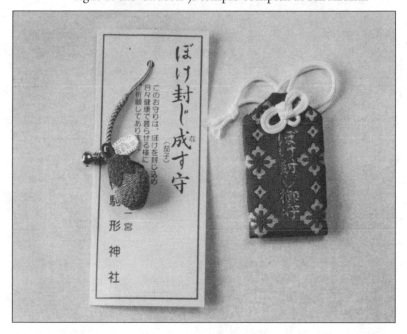

ple and how this differs from the protection one receives from one's parents, one woman stated, "Well, we don't consult with the *kami-sama*. But, again, sometimes I do talk at the *kamidana* [god shelf]." Eventually, after a bit of thought, she equated protection given by the *kami* with the notion that humans are cared for by nature (*shizen*), without specifying exactly how that protection or care is enacted beyond the abstract notion that humans are part of and dependent upon nature—or in her words, "if there's no nature, we're dead." Other informants conceptualized protection in more concrete ways, particularly in relation to the ancestors who are often presented as watching over the world of the living, a point I will discuss in more detail in the next chapter. Regardless of the nature of how protection is conceptualized, individuals purchase *omamori* to protect themselves and others from misfortune, as well as to insure success or health.

Like the *torii* at Benkei-dō, the ubiquity of *omamori* at Chūson-ji points out the lack of concern Japanese have for the divisions between Shintō and Buddhist sacred objects and practices. Normally, *omamori* are found at Shintō shrines, rather than at Buddhist temples, although, as the case of Chūson-ji shows, this is by no means universal. Like the ambiguities that lie within the notion of sectarian association of religious objects and sacred spaces, the specific purpose of *omamori* is difficult to identify. One Shintō priest in Akita explained the purpose of *omamori* as follows: "you should buy *omamori* for health [*kenkō*] if you are already healthy to maintain that health and for sickness [*byōki*] if you are sick and want to recover. In each case, you should keep the *omamori* close to your person, touching your body and should buy a new one each year." Japanese do, in general, keep *omamori* close to their person if they choose to have one, sometimes hooking one to a backpack or carrying one in a pocket or purse.

But people do not necessarily put a great deal of stock in the power of the *omamori*, even while purchasing them regularly. During a discussion with a group of six people in Akita about religious practice, I asked if any of them had ever purchased *omamori* and if so, why. Most had, but the reasons why were varied, including some who had purchased them as good luck charms or souvenirs and one woman who said that she collected them because they are attractive. Another woman among the group noted the comodification of *omamori*, describing the sale of *omamori* at shrines and temples as a business. Two of the women in the group were actually carrying *omamori* in their purses and one had one hanging in her car. One woman stated: "My *omamori* helps to keep me healthy and peaceful. Or at least it helps in a psychological sense. When I see the *omamori* I feel better if I believe it will help." A young man in the group who was in his twenties stated that he had never bought an *omamori* for himself, but when he was young he received them as gifts from his grandparents for safety and to prevent accident. From his perspective, *omamori* is something to be given to others, rather than something one purchases for oneself, as a way of showing that one cares about the other person. He thought that it might represent a sign of affection in that people buy them for those whom they care about and about whose health they are concerned. Or as a woman in the group stated, "it is good for health or luck. It is a feeling that I am loved by somebody and can help us feel better and control our health. It is for affection." And another man stated, "maybe *omamori* are a way of removing ourselves from cynicism."

More important than the spiritual power of *omamori* is the thought associated with giving or receiving one. As one man in his early twenties explained about the only *omamori* he has:

> My father bought it for me for my senior high school entrance examination. I was glad to get it, because it showed my father's feelings, my father's concern—this made me happy. But I didn't bring it with me to the test. I hung it up on my wall, where it is to this day. I cannot ever throw it away, because if I did, I would feel bad [*kimochi warui*].[11]

At the temple hall at Hiraizumi in which the deity (*hotoke*) Yakushi Nyōrai is enshrined, one can purchase *omamori* with the hiragana symbol for the sound *mě* on the front of it, which is also the sound used for the word for eyes. According to a woman working at this temple hall, the deity enshrined there is helpful in protecting (*mamoru*) one's eyes. When I asked her if I could improve my own eyesight by doing *omairi* there, she was hesitant and then said, "I have heard of people with eye problems getting better after doing *omairi* here." Although specifically associated with eyes, along the front of the sales counter at this temple hall banners announce the particular *omamori* one can buy and the purpose of each one: *me-*

mamori for the eyes, *atama-mamori* for the head/brain, *ashikoshi-mamori* for the legs and lower back, *chōju-mamori* for a long life, *kodomo-mamori* for fertility/children, and *boke-mamori* to prevent senility. The prices of these *omamori* range from ¥300 to ¥500, depending upon the design and composition of the object (some are simply silk pouches and some have metal and plastic parts), and the particular *omamori* found at the various temple halls at Chūson-ji are similar (often identical) to those found at sacred sites in other parts of Japan.

At the center of the religious complex is the main hall known as Chūson-ji. One enters through a large gate into an open area across from which is the large main temple building. The air is filled with the smell of burning incense and one can hear the occasional ring of the large bell to one side of the area or the melodic chants of priests from inside the main building. To the right there are stalls selling many of the religious objects also found at the other stalls, but there is an additional one selling Japanese tea that is supposed to be good for health. There are no *omamori* at these stalls, instead one finds sutras, prayer beads, statuary for one's family altar, and other objects available for purchase from a monk seated behind the display table. The presence of a monk at this stall is unlike the others at the religious complex that are invariably occupied by middle-aged women.

In the middle of the open area, there is a large caldron-shaped incense burner (*kōro*) covered by a small roof. This is filled with ashes and is used for burning incense that can be bought at one of the nearby stalls. Next to the caldron, there is a stone basin into which water pours constantly, and which is used as a means of purifying oneself prior to doing *omairi* in front of the temple building by symbolically removing the pollution of the outside, non-sacred space beyond the temple gates (cf. Ohnuki-Tierney 1984). There are cups with long handles placed on the rock and these are used to dip water, which is then washed over each hand and either touched to one's lips or taken in the mouth and then spit out. One can easily overestimate the religious significance of purification in this context. It is not unusual for people to do *omairi* directly, without purifying themselves first, and it is routine to see tourists, particularly middle-school children on fieldtrips, gathered around and drinking the cool water to refresh themselves on a hot day.

In the large open area in front of the temple building, one also can find benches for taking a rest and to the left of the entrance there is a tall rack on which have been hung hundreds of *ema* (which I will discuss in detail below), small wooden tablets that are used to write messages to the *kami* or Buddhist deities. During most of my trips to Chūson-ji, this rack had been located directly in front of the main temple hall, however, in the summer of 2002, it had been moved to the left of the main entrance.

Upon entering this area, people often spend a few minutes admiring the beauty of the building and its surrounding grounds and then head directly to do *omairi*. Styles of *omairi* vary from one person to another. In one case, I observed a woman who came in with an apparent friend. She rinsed her hands and mouth with the water and then went to the front of the temple where she threw some money into the box for collecting offerings, placed her hands together in front of her face, closed her eyes, and remained in that position for more than thirty seconds. She then went to purchase an *ema*, sat down to write her message, and walked across the area to put the *ema* on the rack. She spent a considerable amount of time looking for the proper place to hang the *ema*, finally deciding to place it entirely at the back of several that were hanging from the hooks on the rack.

A few minutes later, a group of middle-school girls and boys, the girls in their dark blue sailor suits and the boys in their black military-style tunics, came into the area and raced to the front of the temple to do *omairi* as a group. Following this, they purchased incense and went to the incense burner to light the incense and place it in the center. The girls were having a great deal of fun running to the large pot, at which they used their hands to waft the smoke from the incense over their heads, an act that is said to be beneficial to improving one's intelligence. As they did this, they said, "make my head/brain good [*atama ga yoku naru*]" and giggled and laughed as they did so. I asked one girl if she thought the smoke would actually help her improve her intelligence and she adamantly replied that she thought it would. As I stood watching the school girls and boys, two women, one in her sixties and the other in her thirties, came up to the caldron and began wafting the smoke over their bodies and saying "to my knee [*ohiza ni*], to my head [*atama ni*], to my feet/legs [*ashi ni*]." I told the women that I had thought the incense smoke was only good for the brain, to which they replied that it was for the health of one's entire body, as well as for each specific part.

Eventually, three of the school girls broke off from the main group and headed for the *ema* rack. They stood for several minutes reading the messages on the *ema*, giggling and joking about the various requests and taking particular interest in a caricature style self-portrait that had been drawn on one. As previously noted, *ema* are wooden tablets that are usually five-sided with a string attached for hanging on a rack at a shrine or temple. Normally, there is a design on one side and on the other there is space on which one can write a message to the deities enshrined at the site where one purchases the *ema*. There are numerous themes and designs in which *ema* are made. Common themes include a picture of the appropriate animal for one's birth year on the Chinese zodiac that is also used in Japan, an arrow pointing at a target, or a Buddha sitting in the lotus position. At one shrine in Mizusawa that is widely known for being beneficial for study, the *ema* are designed in the shape of a large pencil. Both Western and Japanese scholars have been interested in *ema*, especially folklorists (see, for example, Yanagita 1970), and Ian Reader (1991) has given us a very detailed discussion of the history and meanings of *ema* that also briefly addresses the issue of the commodification of religious objects in Japan.

The messages written on *ema* can have considerable variation and there is nothing preventing someone from writing whatever he or she wants. However, they generally fall into the categories of school, health, fertility, love, and general success. Figure 4.9 shows an example of an *ema* that was written at Chūson-ji. To the left, there is space to write one's name and address; to the right there is an open area on which to write the specific desire one wishes to express. The word used to identify this space on the *ema* is *onegai*, which can translate as a desire or as want as in *onegai shimasu*, which is a way to request someone to do that for which one has asked. In Figure 4.9, the author of the *ema* has

Figure 4.9 An example of an *ema* from Chūson-ji. The inscription reads, "to get over the sickness quickly" and gives the name and address of the person who wrote it (which has been deleted to protect the person's identity). (This is approximately six inches across.)

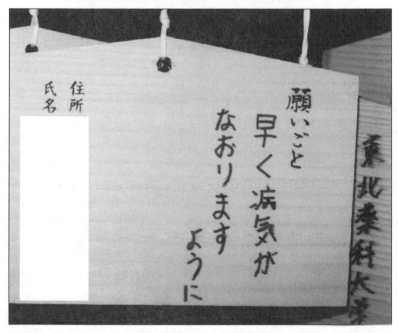

asked for a quick recovery from some unspecified illness. Because Japanese usually refrain from using indefinite articles, it is unclear if the *ema* refers to the author or to someone about whom the author cares.

Other examples from Chūson-ji and other temples and shrines in the area convey some of the variety, and sometimes the sadness, of these messages to the deities. For example, on one *ema* that appeared to be written by a family, the authors request a recovery for their loved one.

May Kayoko get well soon.   *Kayoko hayaku yoku naru yō ni*
Makoto, Keiko, Taka, Mari,   *Makoto, Keiko, Taka, Mari,*
Grandpa, and Grandma   *Ojī-chan, Obā-chan*

Reference to one's family is common on *ema*. The following two are typical examples of *ema* found at Chūson-ji. Both of these request health and safety for the family of the author.

May everyone in the family avoid illness and live in health.	*Kazoku ga mina byōki na dosazu, kenkō de kurasu koto ga dekimasu yō ni*
Wife's safety	*Kanai anzen*

It is also common to find *ema* that request the health of a newborn child. In several *ema* at Chūson-ji, the author indicates the date of birth of the child and then requests that the child have a healthy life.

May the baby be a healthy and bright child. Born: Oct. 31, Heisei 7 (1995)	*Kenkō de akarui ko ni Heisei 7 nen 10 gatsu 31 nichi umare*

One can also find multiple requests on the same *ema*. One example from Chūson-ji requested both the birth of a child and that the author lose weight. In another case, a student requested that he get along well with his friends in junior high school and that he do well in basketball. Love is a particularly common theme and in some cases, such as an *ema* I found at Komagata Jinja in Mizusawa, the author may be very specific in indicating the object of desire.

May I fall in love with X-kun in the class 1-1 in Kamiōkubo Junior High School. Please grant this.	*Kamiōkubo shiritsu chūgaku ichi nen ichi kumi X-kun to ryōomoi ni naremasu yō ni. Onegai itashimasu.*

At Chūson-ji, the majority of *ema* are concerned with maintanence of health, recovery from illness, or insuring the happiness, success, and safety of oneself and one's family. People write *ema* alone, with friends, or with family. It may be done with the serious intent of invoking the power of the deities, or simply as a form of cheap entertainment. As noted above, it is not uncommon for school children on field trips to take great pleasure in reading the various notes on the *ema* at Chūson-ji, suggesting that it is not only entertainment for the writer but also for the potential reader. As Ian Reader notes, the specific focus of *ema* at a particular shrine or temple will often reflect the benefit for which that institution is known, but it does not always work that way. Reader cites statistical data collected by a group of Japanese researchers from Osaka University in which Ishikiri shrine, which is known for healing, actually had more *ema* directed toward education (22 percent) than good health (10 percent) and family safety (7 percent) (Reader 1991:42), although it can be argued that the dividing line between health and family safety may not be particularly clear.

Reader (1991:43) argues that *ema* represent "expressive elements reflecting the all-encompassing nature of Japanese religiosity, in which all human needs and desires are regarded as legitimate issues for which to call upon the spiritual help of the *kami* and buddhas." This clearly sums up one of the main functions of *ema* as a means of expressing concern within the context of the spiritual realm and points out the fact that the emphasis in this form of practice is on pragmatics or securing benefits in this world for oneself and for those to whom one is close. This is often extended beyond the individual to include members of one's family or one's friends and acquaintances.

May I pass the entrance exam for the high school of my first choice. May everybody also pass the exam.	*Shibō taka ni gōkakushimasu yō ni sore kara mina mo issho ni gōkakushimasu yō ni.*

As the junior high school boy who wrote the above *ema* makes clear, while requesting one's own success, one also will often express a desire for the success, health, or happiness of others with whom one is connected.

What I want to stress here is that at the center of the use of *ema* and *omamori* is the idea of well-being, both collective and individual. Talismans and votive tables are used as a way of expressing one's desire that one's family, one's friends, and oneself have productive, happy, and healthy lives in which one's desires are achieved. This should not be interpreted as suggesting that Japanese people view *ema* or other objects such as *omamori* as having magical power. Although some Japanese may believe these objects have magical or other powers, I have found no instances in which people ascribe magical power to *omamori* or *ema*; instead, people typically interpret their use of these objects as having benefits to one's inner-self (one's *kokoro*). Writing an *ema* or keeping an *omamori* in one's purse provides a degree of serenity or comfort. Some of my informants have indicated that they enjoy having an *omamori* simply because they find it aesthetically pleasing and, thus, enjoy having it with them to look at occasionally. Again, use of these objects is connected to individual well-being. Carrying an *omamori* in one's purse or backpack provides a small degree of happiness, or at least a sense of security that one is thinking about the well-being of oneself and the others with whom one interacts. The practice is not a matter of engaging magical powers, but one of keeping individual and collective well-being in mind.

The writing of *ema* and the use of talismans and amulets, unlike other forms of religious practice, are not compartmentalized on the basis of age. People of all ages acquire talismans and visit temples and shrines to do *omairi* and perhaps write an *ema*. Locales such as Chūson-ji have visitors ranging from small children to the very old and many people will purchase a talisman, write an *ema*—and virtually all of them will do *omairi* and make a small money offering at one or more of the temple halls. Certainly, the emphasis on education, particularly success in high school or college entrance exams, encourages young people to engage in this form of ritual practice, even if it is simply a way of making sure that one does everything possible to insure success. But people of all ages regularly purchase or receive talismans and are certain to do *omairi* when they visit a shrine or temple, even if they do not purchase anything to take away with them or purchase an *ema* to hang on the rack.

Smaller temples and shrines will not have talismans and *ema* available for purchase. The main shrine in Kanegasaki, for instance, does not have a full-time priest, thus there usually is no-one there from whom to buy religious objects—although they are made available on special occasions such as the New Year. When one visits a large temple such as Chūson-ji, as noted at the beginning of this section, there are numerous stalls from which one can purchase all manner of religious objects. As noted earlier, the purchase of a talisman, for instance, may be for oneself, but often will be to bring home as a souvenir of the visit. A grandmother may purchase a talisman intended for good health for a sick friend or one for success in study for her grandson preparing for college entrance examinations. Such a talisman serves the dual purpose of being a souvenir of the trip and being a symbol of the concern and love that the giver shows to the recipient.

After writing an *ema* and hanging it, people at the main temple hall at Chūson-ji may pose for pictures and then move onward to look at other parts of the temple complex. At the far end of the main path, there is a large, red *torii* that signifies entrance into another area of the temple complex. Through this gate, one walks along another shaded path, with a large grove of bamboo trees on one side—an uncommon sight in the cold north. At the end of this path is another *torii* directly in front of a large stage for performances of the *nō* theater (*nō butai*). Behind the stage is a Shintō shrine, known as Hakusan-jinja, identifiable by the large rope and bell hanging in front of the entrance where people do *omairi*. In front of the shrine is a large hoop, approximately ten feet in height, made of straw with three paper streamers hanging from the top, middle.

Like at the other temple halls throughout the complex, at Hakusan-jinja there is a booth devoted to selling of talismans and *ema*. I asked the woman behind this counter if there was any special benefit to be gained from doing *omairi* at this shrine and she responded that there is no particular benefit, but that if one goes through the straw hoop that stands in front of the shrine it will cleanse one's inner heart or mind center (*jibun no kokoro o kirei ni shite kureru*). She described passing the hoop as being generally good for one's emotions (*kanjō*) and would bring a good feeling to whomever passes through. To the right of the shrine there is a series of small shrines devoted to each of the signs on the Chinese zodiac where one can do *omairi* and make an offering at the shrine for the year of one's birth.

At a shrine located in Akita City, the centrality of health and well-being was made very clear by a woman who had just finished doing *omairi* in front of the main shrine building. This woman, who was in her fifties or sixties, told me that she will typically go to the shrine when she or a friend is sick, but specifically what she does at the shrine varies in relation to the illness.

> In general, I buy an *omamori* when the illness is not severe and I reserve *ema* for times of greater illness. The cost of the item bought is related to the level of illness. A mild illness will get a less expensive *omamori*; the more extreme the illness, the more the cost of the object that I buy.

For this woman, there is a direct correlation between the level of illness and the amount of money she uses when visiting a shrine. As we chatted, she went on to state that she will put more money in the coin box at the front of the shrine when she is doing *omairi* if the illness in question is more serious. A minor illness will bring a minor amount of money. When I gave her some examples of particular illness, she responded with the following amounts:

common cold = 10 yen to 50 yen

broken bone = around 500 yen

cancer = at least 1,000 and more likely 3,000 to 5,000 yen

Enacting Concern

In exploring different forms of practice used in Japanese religious activity throughout this chapter, I have tried to convey two basic points. First, that we should view Japanese religious activity as being neither Shintō nor Buddhist, but as being ritual without necessary reference to institutional sects. While it is possible to identify connections between particular practices or sacred objects and institutions, there is little concern among most Japanese over the differentiation of Shintō and Buddhism, nor is there a great deal of concern about the specific types of spiritual entities (*kami* or *hotoke*) to which one prays when visiting a temple or shrine. Indeed, I have concluded in numerous discussions on the purposes behind *omairi* and the use of talismans and votive tablets that the emphasis is fundamentally not directed towards the deities. Instead, one does *omairi*, purchases an *omamori*, or writes an *ema* as a means of expressing the interconnectedness of people with the world around them, particularly with the other people, both dead and alive, with whom one has a close relationship. The emphasis is on doing things that express *concern* over the well-being of others; doing *omairi* is a way of showing love, affection, friendship, or simply indicating that one recognizes one's connection to others by thinking about the well-being of other people and enacting that thought through ritual performance.

In other words, Japanese religious activity, rather than being viewed as a means to engage the deities, should be viewed as a means of enacting concern (emotional, obligational, or otherwise) through ritual performance. The temple complex at Chūson-ji, like other sacred spaces, forms a context in which one can engage in ritual activities, in the form of *omairi*, that are aimed at thinking about both the well-being of oneself and one's family and friends and contemplating specific desires, such as the improvement of one's eyes or success in exams. This is true not only in the context of public *omairi*, but also in the context of private *omairi* done in the home at the family *butsudan* or at the *kamidana*. When one does *omairi* at home, one is not simply making an offering to one's ancestors, one is contemplating one's place in the world—having been born from those ancestors— and one is thinking about and remembering a person or people whom one loved deeply, or simply expressing one's caring for another.

One way to think about this is to view Japanese religion as a framework through which people organize their thoughts and emotions about others. It is a way to express the concerns and connections that one has to other people. It expresses the relationship found in what Plath (1980:225) refers to as the convoy of consociates to whom one is closely connected through cumulative interactions and experiences that generate bonds of trust and emotional attachments. In the example cited earlier in this chapter, in which people bring ice cream for a deceased friend for whom this was a favorite food, one person who did this explained it in this way: "the ice cream isn't exactly for the dead person, it is for his wife. It shows that I am concerned about her and thinking about her and recognize her loss." In short, the ice cream is a symbol of the caring and concern she feels for the wife of the man who died. By bringing something he liked when he was alive, this symbolically represents those emotions and brings awareness of the fact that her loss has not been forgotten. Japanese religious activity is far less about deities and powers than it is about concern and well-being. Shrines, temples, *butsudan*, and *kamidana* are contexts at which one can ritually structure and express one's emotions.

A great deal has been written to argue that Japanese do not express their emotions publicly, nor do they express them through physical contact as is common in Western societies. I am arguing that *omairi* and other forms of ritualized expression such as purchasing and writing *ema* or giving *omamori* is a form of expressing concern, rather than a form of prayer, per se. These activities are means by which Japanese express their inner feelings through the framework of ritual performance. A mother might never directly say, "I love you" to her son, but will buy him an *omamori* to help him in his preparation for college entrance exams, which effectively conveys the same meaning. A friend may feel helpless at her inability to do anything for her friend battling cancer—writing an *ema* at the local shrine is a way to "do something," a way to enact one's concern in terms of both personal frustration over helplessness and caring for the person facing an illness. Put in the sense that Tillich uses the idea of concern as ultimate, the ultimate concern in Japanese religious activity is the connections one has with others—concern with the living and the dead with whom one interacts in life and death.

Chapter 5

Old Women, Ancestors, and Caregiving

In the long night of autumn
The dead and the living appear indistinguishably
In my dreams.[1]

—Itoh Setsuko

Japanese conceptualize human/deity or living/ancestor relationships in terms of interaction and interdependence in which mutual well-being is protected and maintained through ritual action. Ritual action related to *kami* and ancestors places the expression of emotional bonds into a structured framework of symbolic behavior that signifies human attachment and caring. However, these activities also are perceived as having practical consequences. Some people view *kami* and ancestors as having the potential to directly influence the world of the living in positive and negative ways, and ancestors, in particular, are implicated in the prosperity and success of one's family, which many view as an outgrowth of ancestral beneficence and protection even if no concrete, causal association is necessarily identified (Smith 1974).

Examples of the association of ancestral interest with the success of the living are evident throughout the ethnographic literature on Japanese religious practice. Stewart Guthrie (1988), for example, notes that some members of the "new" religion known as Risshō-kosei-kai comment that memorializing one's ancestors is beneficial because they are both interested and influential in events of the household of the living. By contrast, ancestral neglect runs the risk of bringing misfortune, such as financial ruin, illness, or accident, upon the family. Within some new religions, proper practice of rituals associated with ancestor veneration is conceptualized as a prescription that has the potential to cure personal and familial ailments and also forms a kind of preventive "medicine" directed toward the avoidance of disaster and illness (Guthrie 1988, Davis 1980). In Byron Earhart's detailed discussion of the new religion known as Gedatsu-kai, he quotes one informant who draws a clear association with illness, misfortune, and the ancestors:

> But as I said before, there was sickness in the family, and other people were trying to help us. When we wondered about the reason [for the sickness], my wife and relatives said that it was some offense against the ancestors or the kami (Earhart 1989:47). (Brackets in original.)

Earhart's informant goes on to explain that his mother-in-law told him that he should go and pay his respects to his ancestors in a distant city and that his failure to visit their memorial stone meant that he had "abandoned" his ancestors. This was interpreted by religious leaders as the cause of their difficulties; the remedy coming in a special ritual treatment of the neglected ancestors to eliminate their condition as *muenbotoke*, or wandering spirits (1989:47–49). Indeed, the approach to solving the problems experienced by Earhart's informant follow a pattern of diagnosis and cure—the neglected ancestors being restored to a state of well-being through expression of concern by living family members via proper ritual observance.

Although ideas about the manner in which ancestors operate in the living world are often ambiguous, if even considered at all, ancestral concern is typically interpreted in terms of the idea that one is always being watched over and protected by one's ancestors. When two women in their seventies were asked, "Do you think your grandma protects you?", they quickly responded "*mite ite kureru*" and "*mamotte kureru*," both of which indicate being protected in the sense of being watched over.[2] Hikaru Suzuki argues that this conceptualization of the ancestors as protectors may be waning in contemporary society. She sees a shift away from traditional veneration of household ancestors to a more abstract memorialism of the ancestors through offerings. Contermporary funerary practices such as spreading the ashes of the deceased, rather than burial of the ashes in the family grave, are an indication of a movement "in the direction of the personal celebration of the deceased's life as a non-specific 'antecedent', separate from the household ancestors, the continuation of the household or becoming an ancestor for the descendants" (Suzuki 1998:185). Suzuki argues that, associated with this shift to a more personal orientation to memorialization, the relationship between the dead and the living is becoming increasingly horizontal, rather than vertical. There is less concern about specific power of the ancestors over the living.

While this trend is an important one to consider the extent of the change may be reflected generationally—in relation to the elderly, at least, the tutelary power of the ancestors over their descendants continues to be important. If Suzuki is correct, this may well be a cohort effect—as the current elder population dies out, the power of the ancestors may die with it. However, an alternative explanation is that as people age and grow closer themselves to becoming ancestors, the power of the ancestors becomes increasingly visceral. For many elderly, particularly elder women,[3] the ancestors are not simply passive observers of the living world. They can and do take an active role in warning the living of impending problems or showing general concern about the world of the living by appearing in dreams.[4]

Before moving on, I want to emphasize that my interest here does not lie in the presentation or the interpretation of the dreams these informants discussed.[5] Rather, I am interested in my informants' interpretation of their ancestral dream experiences and their conceptualizations of the significance of such experiences. In many cases, the recollections of dreams are quite short; all of the informants interviewed discussed dreams that had happened in the past, or indicated that the dreams themselves were never particularly detailed. In some cases, informants did not remember the specific circumstances in which the dream had occurred, but were certain that dreams in which

ancestors appeared had been part of their experience. More important than the specific content of the dreams is the fact that these
dream experiences are presented as a common part of personal memory claims that are used to indicate that the ancestors are directly involved in the world of the living. As a personal memory claim, these
dreams can be understood as bodily and embodied linkages between
the living and dead that index the bi-directionality of concern.[6]

The tendency of older women in particular to contextualize these
dream experiences in terms of concern and protection is significant,
because it reflects Japanese conceptualizations of women as the individuals primarily responsible for providing care and managing health
matters within the domestic sphere. Although adult women at any
age may carry this responsibility, as women enter into middle and old
age, they often take on the role of caretaker of the collective well-
being of the family and become the primary individuals responsible
for expressing concern in relation to the well-being of both living and
dead family members. Older women often interpret the appearance
of ancestors in their dreams as a signal that the ever-watching ancestors are concerned and that something is amiss in the world of the
living.[7] I will return to this point and a more detailed discussion of
the role of women as "healers" within the family at the end of this
chapter, but for now I want to turn to the discussion of specific
dreams.[8]

Dreams and the Departed

Nara Yai is a 65 year-old woman living in a three-generation family consisting of her eldest son, his wife, and their two children in the
hamlet known as Yamada discussed in chapter 4. Always ready to
show her sharp wit and warm smile, Nara is a busy woman, spending much of her time caring for her grandchildren after school and
managing many of the activities of the household, including daily ancestor veneration. Nara and I discussed her experiences of dream visitation while sitting in the entryway of her house, sipping iced tea and
enjoying the summer breeze—a refreshing break from the intense

humidity of summer in Akita Prefecture. For Nara, "the ancestors protect the family (*ie*), but more than that, they are *asked* to protect the family." It is interesting that in Nara 's comments, the element of need is presented as being stronger for the living than the dead, and whatever the ancestors provide in terms of protection is at the request of the living. In this simple statement, she makes it clear that it is the living who *petition* the dead for protection and it is out of beneficence that the dead provide it, rather than out of obligation. Nara 's comments raise the point that while the relationship between the living and dead is reciprocal, it is also asymmetrical: the responsibility for protecting the stem-family rests primarily with the living, who petition the dead for whatever help they may provide. Other informants offered similar comments that indicate the asymmetrical relationship of the living and dead. Morita Hiroshi, a retired schoolteacher in his mid-sixties whose narrative I have discussed elsewhere (Traphagan 2000a:57) put it this way:

> In terms of responsibility of the successor [the child who is normally charged with primary responsibility for caring for the ancestors], I think that it is important to protect [*mamoru*] the stem-family [*ie*]. It would be unfortunate if my stem-family came to die. Thus, someone needs to protect and care for the house, family, garden, rice fields, grave, and ancestors. If you give up the responsibility as successor, everything will come apart—all of those things and the family will expire.

Although the responsibilities of the successor are an important element in Morita's comments, the potential harm to the ancestors by failing to carry out this responsibility (and by extension the potential for harm to come to the living) is an additional motivation for enacting ancestor rituals. Morita explained that should the successor or other family members fail to provide for the ancestors through ritual memorialization, he worried that the ancestral spirits might become wandering spirits in the same way that Earhardt's informant, discussed above, experienced this outcome of failing to carry out one's ritual and filial responsibilities. As I noted earlier, the *muenbotoke* condition arises as a result of neglect by one's descendants—a failure of the living to ritually express their concern for the well-being of their predecessors.

Morita's wife, also present during the conversation, went on to state that she asks the ancestors to protect their family, and is convinced that they are able to actively provide protection, a point that started a somewhat heated disagreement among the couple. Mr. Morita argued that the ancestors do not respond to the specific requests of the living. Instead, their presence provides a vague, generalized protection of the stem-family. In contrast, Mrs. Morita stated that she directly asks the ancestors for protection when she does *omairi* at the family altar: "When my husband is away, particularly when he has traveled overseas, I go to the altar and ask the ancestors to watch over him and make sure that he gets home safely." Following this comment by Mrs. Morita, Mr. Morita scoffed and rather emphatically stated that requesting specific protection from the ancestors is useless because they cannot intervene directly. This does not mean that performing *omairi* is useless in Mr. Morita's mind. Indeed, he commented that one does *omairi* for the personal benefit that comes from thinking about and showing concern for one's ancestors: "although you do not get help, it is good to do *omairi* from a personal perspective in terms of one's *kokoro* [center, heart, mind]. You do *omairi* for yourself and your own *kokoro*. But it is useless for asking for things in particular" (Traphagan 2000a:57).

The debate between Mr. and Mrs. Morita is a good indication of the fact that there is no consensus on whether or not ancestors involve themselves directly in the world of the living—personal experience and beliefs play a major role in how people construct their conceptualization of ancestral involvement in the living family. There is, however, general agreement that it is important for the living to involve themselves in providing ritual care for the deceased. Regardless of how people conceptualize the involvement of the dead in the world of the living, or the potential of the dead to become *muenbotoke*, there is widespread agreement among Japanese that one has a responsibility to care for one's ancestors.

It is interesting that, at least among the people with whom I have discussed this issue, women are more likely to indicate that the dead have the power to actively influence the lives of their descendants. Indeed, it was within the context of asking individuals about how the ancestors engage the living world that women, in particular, expressed this involvement in terms of specific dream experiences. For example, Nara explained that she knows that her ancestors are protecting the family because they appear in dreams when problems arise that require the members of the living family to act. Furthermore, as a warning that there is a problem that requires attention, an ancestor will appear in a dream. Nara went on to discuss a specific dream that she had on repeated occasions in which Obā-chan (her deceased, co-resident mother-in-law) appeared. The dream consisted simply of Obā-chan working in the garden, an image that Nara associated with her mother-in-law who spent much of her time in later life weeding and doing other garden work. As Nara explained it, when this dream occurs, Obā-chan does not speak, but merely appears in the familiar guise of work. The significance Nara places in this dream lies in its indication that her mother-in-law is continuing to watch over her from the grave—while she has departed the world of the living, she continues to be concerned about the well-being of her descendants.

Dreams in which a relative appears but does not speak represent the basic plot of virtually all of the ancestral dreams described by the women and men with whom I spoke. This plot-line typically involved the appearance of a close relative, often the deceased grandmother of an extended family, carrying out some form of work that she commonly did while alive, but without any direct action or verbalization aimed at the dreamer or her family. Indeed, among those with whom I have discussed these dream experiences, there is a widely held belief that rather than speaking directly to the living in dreams, ancestors simply appear—in the event that an ancestor does speak in a dream it is to be interpreted negatively, although the specific implications were invariably left vague. Indeed, the key element in Nara's dream, and in the other dream experiences discussed by these older women and men, was the appearance of the ancestor him or herself; the interpretation of why the ancestor appeared was left entirely up to the individual who experienced the dream, a fact that reinforces the idea mentioned by Nara that the onus of responsibility for action rests primarily on the living.

In the case of Nara, her ancestral dream meant that there was something threatening the health of her family. She said, "the dream meant that we need to take care of my/our body(ies) [*karada o daiji ni*]," referring to herself and her family. The Japanese Nara uses leaves it vague as to the specific person or people to whom she is referring, because, as is common in Japanese, she does not use a definite article. However, she goes on to situate the meaning of this and other similar dreams she had experienced in terms of familial well-being: "I think, when the ancestors show up in a dream, it means that they are in some way worrying about the family."[9] Nara's interpretation of the dream as indicating her ancestor's concern over the well-being of the family is a theme that arose frequently enough that at times it seemed almost clichéd.

Suzuki Aiko (60), expressing sentiments about her dream experiences that were quite similar to those of Nara, stated that she has had repeated dreams in which her ancestors appeared, the occurrence of which she always interprets as a warning.

> I have dreams in which my ancestors, particularly my mother-in-law, come and tell me that I should be careful [*ki o tsukeru*]. I see my mother-in-law's face or see her out working in the fields in these dreams. The dreams are not very specific, but there is a sense from them that the family should take extra care. I then tell my family about the dream and that they should take care.

Like Nara, Suzuki states that she has had repeated experiences of dreams in which her ancestors, specifically her mother-in-law, appear. In each case, she interprets these in terms of ancestral concern about the world of the living family—when an ancestor appears, she interprets the dream as indicating the need for her family to take special care or to take precautions for something unexpected. Although ambiguous in terms of the content of the danger that lies ahead, Suzuki conveys her awareness of ancestral concern to her family each time such a dream occurs. While her family may choose to respond to or ignore the information she conveys—indeed, she did not indicate that the family typically would embark upon particular precautionary activities beyond continued ritual practice, sometimes extending involvement to more members of the family—her possession of information related to ancestral concern places her in a medium-like position between the living and dead. Among the members of her household, Nara is the one who conveys, ambiguous as it may be, concern that has arisen among the ancestors about the living family and that the family members are in some way at risk.

For Oikawa Keiko, who was 72 at the time of our conversation, the appearance of ancestors in dreams is not a warning, but is a clear indication of concern, typically happening after something has gone wrong. Much of Oikawa's relationship to her ancestors revolves around the idea that they can provide some form of protection. She indicated that when she does *omairi*, "Every day when I pray [*ogamu*], I say, 'may my family be healthy' [*kazoku genki de iraremasu yō ni*]." Although she stated that her memory of the specific details about dreams in which her ancestors had appeared was not clear, she was certain that they had appeared and that their appearance arose when something negative had happened to a member of the family or the family as a whole.

> I have seen my ancestors in dreams. I think it has been Grandma or Grandpa [in-laws]. When something happens, I am likely to see them in my dreams. For example, if someone in the family has an accident, they appear. When I think of the ancestors, there is a feeling that I should take care [*ki o tsukete*]. I think they are protecting me.

It is worth noting that in Oikawa's case, visitations by "spirits" were not limited to her ancestors nor to the experience of dreaming; she also indicated an instance in which a *kami* appeared in the alcove (*tokonoma*) next to the family altar. At the time she experienced this, she also had an unusual encounter with a candle that had been burning on the altar—the candle had burned most of the way down and when she picked it up, flame shot from one side. She said that when this happened, "I wondered if I should take the candle somewhere to pray, such as to a shrine or temple, but I wasn't sure so I just put it in the alcove." For the next three days, she said, the *kami* appeared in the alcove (the specifics of what exactly she meant by this were never clear in our conversations), after which there was a fire in the house of her next-door neighbor. In retrospect, she interpreted this entire experience as a warning that something was going to happen and that there was an indexical link to the fire of the candle and to the burning of the neighbor's house.

The examples of these women are representative of a theme that arose frequently in discussions concerning the nature of ancestral protection and the experience of ancestral visitation in dreams. At least among older women, there is a tendency to view one's ancestors as not simply watching over, but as having some degree of agency in relation to the world of the living.[10] More specifically, the recently departed seem to take on a role of maintaining close watch over the living family and of showing ancestral concern when the need arises. Indeed, for virtually all of the women who had dream experiences in which ancestors appeared, it was either their mother-in-law or natal mother who appeared in the dreams. This is not surprising; one would expect that these dreams would involve the recently departed—those whom one remembers, misses, and continues to love and care for in a direct way. But the fact that it was recently departed women who most often were described as appearing in dreams, and that it was elder women who were most likely to discuss these types of dream experiences is instructive and, perhaps, predictable given the emphasis in Japanese culture on the idea that domestic caregiving is fundamentally conceptualized as a feminine role.

Older Women and Concern

The appearance of ancestors in the dreams of the women cited above indexes Japanese notions of continuity between the realms of the living and the dead in terms of experience and need. As Emiko Ohnuki-Tierney argues, through bringing ancestors into daily life via ritual performance, Japanese people symbolically generate a framework in which death is not set apart from human life; death is not a pathological state set against a norm of life (and health) (1984:71).

Notions of continuity and balance are evident not only in notions about the nature of life and death, but also in ideas about health and illness and fortune and misfortune.

In terms of health and illness, more than emphasizing an idealized "healthy" or "normal" body juxtaposed against a diseased body, Japanese emphasize balance. In classical writings on *kanpō* (East Asian medicine), disease is viewed as becoming manifest through an imbalance in the body, the causes of which can be either external or internal, a perspective that is carried into the present within the context of East Asian medical practices (Lock 1980:37–38). The aim of therapeutic actions on the part of patients and health practitioners (often using herbal medicines, acupuncture, etc.) is not restoration of perfect health to an anomalous body that has been dislodged from the norm of health. As Lock states, "[h]ealth and ill-health are both seen as natural and as part of a continuum and are not viewed as a dichotomy" (Lock 1980:43). As such, therapeutic actions on the part of patients and health practitioners are not aimed at dominating and eliminating the debilitating forces of nature—disease and aging—that remove the body from its normal state of perfect health. Rather, the aim is the restoration of balance both internally and between oneself and the milieu in which one lives. Health is achieved by adapting to the external and internal forces that can disrupt balance within a body and among the body and the milieu in which it exists, rather than through the elimination of pathogenic forces.[11]

The two central points here are that: (1) the idea of illness as an anomalous state of the body is not necessarily accepted; and (2) the idea that the transition from life to death alleviates one's potential for suffering, or removes one from the vicissitudes of illness and misfortune (and Ohnuki-Tierny includes pollution, as well) does not obtain for Japanese. If we think back to the *tanka* poem by Itoh Setsuko cited at the beginning of this chapter, there is a sense in which, at least in the world of dreams, there is no distinction between the living and the dead. While this literary allusion should not be taken as necessarily representative of Japanese ideas about dreams or about the relationship between living and dead, it at least can be interpreted as indexing Japanese sensibilities about the fuzziness between these worlds.

Both the living and the dead are subject to the forces of illness and misfortune. While, as Lock (1980) shows, specialized medical practitioners of East Asian medicine work with the ill to restore balance, practitioners of cosmopolitan biomedicine are less inclined to follow this approach. And, indeed, most Japanese make extensive use of cosmopolitan biomedicine when faced with illness or functional decline associated with aging, although it is common for older people to supplement biomedical medicine with herbal and other forms of medicine associated with traditional East Asian approaches to healing. Nonetheless, the concept of maintaining balance to ensure health and well-being remains important for Japanese and the central figures in practices associated with maintaining life-balance are women. Not only is balance important in terms of the individual, but it also is important in terms of the relationship between the living and the dead. It is this point I wish to focus upon here.

Within the context of the domestic sphere, the maternal, caring role of women is extended in multiple directions, incorporating concern for one's children, and in multigenerational families, at least, one's parents or in-laws. In households such as those of the women discussed above, in which there are deceased members and, thus, a family altar, this caring role is also directed towards the predecessors of the household. For these women, dreams are one context in which the continuity between the ancestral world and the living world is expressed and through which, in a way similar to what Kerns (1997:5) finds among Black Carib women in the West Indies, older women sustain social order through expressing concern for their families.[12]

Indeed, it is common that elder women are the family members who have main responsibility for carrying out ancestor-related rituals on a daily basis. While surveying males and females over the age of 65 from 52 households in Kanegasaki in 1996, I found that all but eight respondents indicated that either they themselves or their spouse were the members of the household primarily responsible for conducting daily *omairi*. Furthermore, although anyone in the household may at any time make offerings or pray (the word used in the questionnaire was *ogamu*) at the family altar, it is instructive that most (85 percent) of the respondents in this questionnaire indicated that it was the eldest generation in the household, and particularly elder women, who were most involved in daily veneration practices.[13]

Given that the maternal role extends to all married women in the household and that anyone can participate in ancestor-related rituals, one may ask why ritual action associated with the ancestors is closely associated with elder women. Discussing the transfer of knowledge related to rituals associated with ancestor veneration, Robert J. Smith argues that because older women often take more interest in religious and ritual affairs, they are the logical choice to convey information about the ancestors to other family members, particularly to children. According to Smith, because women have longer life expectancies than men, "the grandmother, where there is one, is usually the oldest household member" (Smith 1974:120). Smith's premise that the long life expectancy of women contributes to their having significant roles in conveying religious knowledge to younger generations seems questionable on the grounds that in many cases long life can also mean disability and, as discussed in chapter 3, considerable difficulties in communicating with younger generations. However, the idea that the elderly, and particularly elderly women, are the closest link with the ancestors because they, more than anyone else in the family, knew the people memorialized in the altar is an important insight in relation to understanding the religious and spiritual roles of individuals in a household and how these roles change over time.

Considering the above narratives, it is clear that knowledge of the deceased intensifies the relationship between living and dead. If we return to the case of Oikawa Hiroko from chapter 4, in her narrative she clearly indicates how specific events in her life changed the manner in which she experiences the act of doing *omairi*. The death of her mother-in-law changed her relationship to the ancestors and infused the experience of doing *omairi* with emotional content it had previously lacked. The idea that the experience of *omairi*, and the relationship to the ancestors, changes over the lifecourse is one that was raised frequently by both men and women.

Awano Erika, who was in her mid-thirties when we spoke, also indicated that the death of a loved one stimulated regular involvement with ancestor rituals:

> When my mother died, my father faithfully brought offerings in the morning and evening to the family altar for her. He did this while his emotions were still strong for her. But after about a year, he stopped doing this so regularly.

This example suggests that for Japanese, religious ritual activity in later life, rather than being connected to aging per se, is tied to the fact that the elderly are more likely to have intimate knowledge of someone who has died—specifically a family member. As one grows older, one is more likely to have known the departed, thus regular involvement in ritual activity is generated not only from obligation but out of emotionally driven desires to remain connected to, and reciprocally involved with, the deceased. The special relationship between the elderly and the departed is also indicated in the fact that in both of the above cases, and in several other narratives I collected, it is the deceased co-resident mother-in-law who appears in the dreams. Following Smith's insight into the connection between the elderly and the departed, this makes sense because of all the deceased members of the household, it is the mother-in-law with whom a co-resident woman (daughter-in-law) is most likely to have had the closest and most frequent interaction. Smith notes that women—those who are wives of the head of household or the grandmother—in households with extended families often have responsibility for the care of the memorial tablets that symbolically represent the dead, and for providing daily offerings of food and drink to the ancestors (although this is by no means universal) (Smith 1974:119).

While it is reasonable to explain the importance of older women in ancestor-related rituals as being an outgrowth of their nearness to the dead, here I want to explore another possible explanation. Throughout this chapter, I have organized my thoughts around the idea that the centrality of elder women in ancestor-related ritual practice is closely connected with Japanese tendencies to define women's roles in terms of both domesticity and caring (cf. Lebra 1986, see also Imamura 1987). From early on in their married lives, women in Japanese society are associated with various forms of care provision. Mothers are expected to devote virtually their entire attention to raising and caring for children, often at the expense of their personal interests and desires.

As Takie Lebra notes, in many cases the center of motherhood is associated with the concept of *ikigai* (which I discussed in relation to aging in chapter 4). Women often refer to their children as their *ikigai*, and a "woman's sexual identity, which predominated her earlier life stage [pre childbirth], is overshadowed by her maternal preoccupation" (Lebra 1986:298). By contrast, participation of men in child-rearing tends toward bipolarity, with either active involvement or virtually no involvement in the lives of their children. The latter is considerably more common than the former (Lebra 1986:179). In later life, when a family member is stricken with terminal illness or elder immediate family members become too frail to care for themselves, women are almost invariably the ones expected to provide most of the daily care—if the children have already grown and moved out, the emphasis on caregiving moves from the children to the elder generation, "whereby she comes to hold a pivotal role as... care-taker for her old parents or parents-in-law as well as her offspring" (Lebra 1986:298).[14] If children are still at home, she is likely to be expected to provide care and attention for both generations (as well as for her husband when needed).

This construction of a woman's identity *qua* caregiver often becomes central even if it is at the expense of a woman's career or pursuit of her own interests. Ariyoshi Sawako's novel *Kōkotsu no Hito* (1972, 1987) provides a particularly poignant example of the idea that not only are women the primary caregivers, but, in fact, their own value is largely expressed in terms of the caregiver role. In the story, middle-aged Akiko struggles to care for her father-in-law, who becomes increasingly debilitated and difficult to care for as a result of senile dementia (*boke*). She deals with helping him to the bathroom, washing him, stopping him from urinating outside, changing diapers, and numerous other symptoms and outcomes associated with dementia, while at the same time keeping her job as a typist. Lacking help from her husband and being unable to secure help from social service organizations she is forced to quit her job. The climax of the novel occurs when she resolves to devote herself completely to caring for her father-in-law:

> All these months she had hated every minute she had had to spend looking after her father-in-law. But, starting today, she vowed to prolong his life for as long as she possibly could, knowing in her heart that she was the only one in the family who was able to do so (Ariyoshi 1987:187).

In the end, Akiko finds herself in the realization that she alone, as the only woman in her household, is able to provide care to her elder father-in-law, ultimately telling a friend that it is her "duty to take good care of Grandpa" (Ariyoshi 1987:188).

The idea that it is a woman's duty to care for others and that it is she, alone, who can provide care is widely accepted in Japanese society. Indeed, between 85 and 90 percent of all long-term care givers in Japan are women, and most of these are relatives, either daughters, daughters-in-law, or wives (Lock 1993:123; Long 1997, 2003; Harris, Long, Fujii 1998). This emphasis on the caregiver role is closely associated with Japanese conceptualizations of femininity as expressed through the idea of *onna rashisa* or womanly behavior, which can include proper use of feminine language, humbleness, neatness, and proper handling of the body (in accord with notions of elegance), and a focus of one's identity on concern for others (Lock 1993:96). In Lock's work on menopause in Japan, she quotes one woman who states that child rearing is a woman's primary function and that "her body is not her own; it's meant for leaving descendants" (1993:98). This underscores the notion that, at least in terms of the discourse on femininity in Japan, there is a sense in which the conceptualization of the feminine role is closely tied to the serving of others. Of course, many women do not adhere to this conceptualization of femininity and some women actively resist it. However, the association of the feminine role with caring for or serving others can be found in a wide variety of contexts, ranging from the hostess clubs described by Allison (1994) to the corporate offices described by Ogasawara (1998) to the home context discussed by Rice (2001).

That women should be primarily responsible for providing "care" in all of the ways made manifest within a family is a notion that is rarely contested in Japanese society. Lock points out that when asked to discuss caring for elders, although all of her informants agreed that it was difficult work, "there was almost no argument that close female relatives should be primarily responsible" for providing care (1993:72). Kondo notes that at times women working in the corporate world, at least part-timers, extend the mother role to the context of work by taking on the caregiver role vis-à-vis men in the company (Kondo 1990:295). She argues that by taking on the mother role, they are able to extend some degree of power over the males with whom they interact, thus increasing their importance in the company. For Kondo, the role of caregiver, "or the one who indulges the selfish whims of another (the amayakasu position)" (1990:295–296) is in fact a superordinate position in which one individual, usually a person in a position of superiority such as a parent or boss, can claim and exert power over others (subordinates). At times this relationship can be reversed as a person in a subordinate role takes on the position of providing indulgence to others.

While the conditions of context that Kondo describes are very different from those within the households discussed here, her basic insight, that subordinates can claim power over otherwise superior individuals through enacting the caregiver role is relevant to the discussion. In chapter 3, I noted that many older people, particularly those living in rural areas, view themselves as isolated from contemporary society. As one woman in her eighties who was living in a three-generation household stated, "We all have our own rooms, separate televisions, and eat at separate times. It's as though we live in separate houses" (for a very similar comment by another older informant, see Traphagan 2000a:180). It is not at all uncommon to hear older people describe themselves and their generation as *furui* meaning old and out-dated or obsolete. Separated from the context of contemporary life, as a woman living in a multi-generation family ages she may become removed from the mainstream life of the family when her son's wife takes on the primary caregiver role towards her children and anticipates providing care to her in-laws. For the elder woman living in a multigenerational household, the central maternal/female role of caregiver is transferred to her daughter or daughter-in-law (depending upon which one with whom she is living).

Older women not living in multigenerational households have different experiences. Single generation elderly households are becoming increasingly common throughout Japan and in these situations a woman may continue to carry on the caregiver role if her husband becomes ill; of course, this can be reversed in the event that the woman becomes ill. And the number of older women living alone has also increased—a living situation that many of my older female informants have indicated they greatly enjoy because they are free from the expectations associated with the caregiver role. Indeed, data from the Ministry of Public Management, Home Affairs, Posts, and Telecommunications show that elder-only households in general and single elder households have been increasing in number for several decades (http://www.stat.go.jp/english/data/nenkan/1431-02.htm). As of 2000, approximately 20 percent of all elder households were single elder and 26 percent elder couple households (see Figure 5.1), meaning that elder-only households represented nearly half of all households in which there was a person over the age of sixty-five (http://www.stat.go.jp/english/data/nenkanzuhyou/b0219000.xls).

While the demographic characteristics of age distribution in relation to household composition is changing in Japan, the relationship between older women and the ancestors remains one of great importance, particularly in multi-generation households, which still represent more than half of those in which elderly Japanese live. Takie Lebra argues that aged women sustain themselves "by an intensified identification with the ancestors, or dead members, of the house" (1986:289). The older woman "waits for *omukae* [literally, to be taken away] to have 'reunion' with the dead" (1986:289). Lebra goes on to describe the role of the elder woman as that of "household priestess," a role that is transferred from the elder woman to her daughter-in-law, in multigeneration families, as the older woman conveys the importance of caring for the ancestors (herself soon to become one) to

Figure 5.1 Growth in Elder-Only Households, 1980–2000

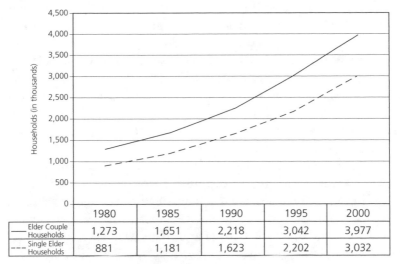

	1980	1985	1990	1995	2000
Elder Couple Households	1,273	1,651	2,218	3,042	3,977
Single Elder Households	881	1,181	1,623	2,202	3,032

Source: Japan Statistical Yearbook, Ministry of Public Management,
Home Affairs, Posts and Telecommunications,
http://www.stat.go.jp/english/data/nenkan/1431-02.htm.

the younger members of the household (1986:289). While I think that describing elder women as household priestesses may well be over-stating their religious role, the importance of women, particularly elder women, in conducting rituals associated with the ancestors cannot be overlooked.

Here, instead of framing this in terms of a "priestess" role, I want to suggest that managing and performing the ritual activities of the family, as well as conveying ancestral dreams, may be one way in which elderly women maintain the caregiver role, and certainly is an expression of the conceptual equation of women with care giving.[15] In the interviews related to ancestor veneration conducted for this book, women's dreams of ancestors were interpreted in terms of well-being, and these women formed the conduit through which ancestral concern about the well-being of the living was conveyed to family members. In this sense, these women express the gendered role of caregiver by linking the living to the dead and thus contributing to the well-being of their families by reporting ancestral concern when it arises. One way to understand the role of these women is to view them as mediums through which ancestral concern is conveyed to the family. An elder woman may have difficulties carrying out the caregiver role in the same way she had earlier in life and she may become the recipient of care by a daughter or daughter-in-law. Nonetheless, this does not mean that she is entirely dislocated from the caregiver role. Rather, she continues to be able to exert agency through caregiving by mediating the worlds of the living and the dead through ritual practice and by conveying the concern of the ancestors about their descendents to the other living members of her family.

In other words, conveying ancestral dreams and carrying out the primary ritual duties associated with ancestor veneration may be one way in which elderly women maintain the caregiver role by being the primary individuals charged with enacting the practice of concern in relation to the ancestors. And as I argued in chapter 2, the well-being of the stem-family, inclusive of the ancestors, is the ultimate concern of Japanese religious practice. Through performance of ancestor-related rituals and through reporting of dream episodes in which ancestors appear, older women take on a central role in the most important element—ancestor veneration—of the total lifecare system that I have described in the previous chapters. It might be argued that these women can be understood as informal "healers" who invoke the aid of the ancestors in maintaining the well-being of the family. While this conceptualization of healer is not intended to imply that by carrying out daily rituals for the ancestors older women are necessarily using spiritual powers to effect cures on the living family members, it can be understood as an extension of the maternal healing/care-giving role as well as a more specialized form of health care provision when specific illness arises within the family.[16]

Chapter 6

Matsuri: *Expressing Collective Concern*

> If you cut a living tree on the neighborhood festival day, you
> will have an accident and be injured.
>
> —(in Brown 1979:227)

In the previous chapters, I explored some of the ways in which individuals participate in ritual practice at sacred sites such as temples,
shrines, and in the home and I argued that *omairi* can be understood
in terms of concern for the well-being of oneself and one's family. In
this chapter, I turn to the public, collective expression of concern
through ritual performance by examining a shrine festival (*matsuri*)
that takes place annually in Kanegasaki. Ashkenazi argues that the
shrine festival he studied in the town of Yuzawa provides entertainment value and a context in which non-festival forms of activity, such
as economic transactions, take place (Ashkenazi 1993:9). These characteristics are evident in the shrine festival in Kanegasaki that I will
discuss in this chapter, but there are two additional features of the
festival that are important to understand for our purposes here. First,
the festival is a public and collective expression of concern for the individuals who comprise the community in which it takes place. Second, the festival symbolically represents the role—the set of assumed
and embodied behaviors associated with one's performative position
in a group—of the elderly as central players in the religious and ritual life of the community. Similar to their role within the household,

within the community the elderly are the caretakers of the expression of (collective) concern and are responsible for managing the process of ritual performances that express that concern. However, in contrast to household-oriented rituals that are primarily the domain of women, in community rituals such as the festival I will discuss here, like the ceremony discussed in the ethnographic vignette that began chapter 1, it is men who manage the ritual performance and through that the expression of concern.[1]

Kabōsai: The Fire Prevention Festival in Kanegasaki

Kabōsai, which translates as fire prevention festival, takes place annually on the third Sunday in April along the narrow streets that twist through the downtown area of Kanegasaki. Local history books produced by the town government, which are largely based on research conducted by local residents, indicate that the impetus behind starting the festival was a series of fires that occurred in the Meiji Era (1868–1912), including a large blaze in 1899 and several smaller fires that destroyed residential and merchant areas of the town. The festival is fashioned after a much older and grander festival that has taken place in neighboring Mizusawa since a major fire destroyed part of that city during the later part of the Edo Period (1600–1867). In Kanegasaki, the festival was first carried out in 1925 in a farming area of town known as Mikajiri. In 1928, people living in the central merchant district of town and the former samurai neighborhoods that are adjacent to the merchant district decided to begin performing the festival. Eventually this area became the festival's focal point for the entire town (Sato et al. 1992:728–729). Figure 6.1 shows a photograph taken in the late-1920's of the group that participated in the festival.

Typical of shrine festivals throughout Japan, *kabōsai* consists of a procession in which sacred objects, including those that house the *kami* of the local Shintō shrine, are carried through the streets (Ashkenazi 1993; Bestor 1989; Schnell 1995). The festival includes

Figure 6.1 Participants in Kabōsai c. 1925

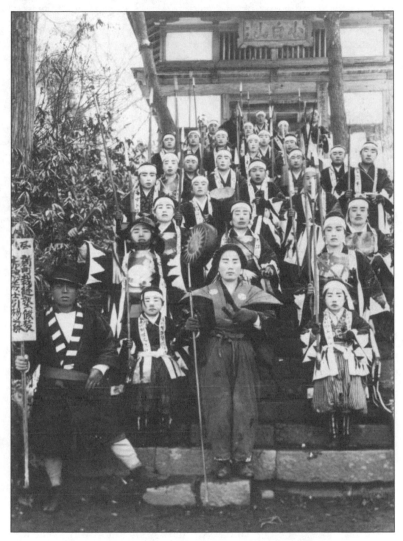

participants from each of the three *ku* or neighborhoods in the downtown area of Kanegasaki—Honchō, Minamimachi, and Jōnai. Honchō, the main merchant district for Kanegasaki, is responsible for

preparation of the *yatai*, a wheeled float that is pulled around the town's streets and carries young girls and, in recent years, boys who are dressed in elaborate kimono. Members of the Honchō Women's Association (*fujinbu*) also participate as dancers in the procession. Minamimachi, a residential area adjacent to Honchō, provides one of two *mikoshi*—portable shrines that are carried or wheeled along the processional route to convey the purificatory power of the *kami* beyond the confines of the main shrine building—that are circulated throughout the neighborhoods during the ritual procession. Minamimachi also sponsors a truck that rides along behind the *mikoshi*. This truck opens like a stage and children from the neighborhood's Children's Association play *taiko* drums at specified stops throughout the procession route.

In 1996, I participated in *kabōsai* as a member of the Young Men's Association for the neighborhood of Minamimachi. In addition to observing the events, I was one of the men who carried the *mikoshi* (see Figure 6.2) throughout the downtown area of Kanegasaki.[2] I will draw specifically on these experiences as I discuss the festival.

At around eight o'clock on the night prior to *kabōsai*, members of the Young Men's Association assemble for a party that goes late into the evening and revolves largely around drinking and socializing. There are congratulatory speeches for having worked hard to prepare for the festival and encouragement for the hard work of carrying the *mikoshi* and managing the festival on the next day. Sushi purchased from a nearby restaurant is served, as well as home-made pickles and snacks such as peanuts to accompany the alcoholic beverages, which include saké, beer, and *shochu* (a strong clear alcohol made with potatoes). Most of the men become inebriated to some degree, and a few become sufficiently drunk to need help in returning home.

Preparations on the day of the *matsuri* begin around 8:00am. Participants gather at the meeting halls (*shūkaijo*) for their respective neighborhoods. Members of the Women's Association and women in the Old Persons Club prepare food throughout the morning, some of which the men consume and some of which will be eaten later in the day. As the time for the festival comes closer, younger men who will carry the *mikoshi* prepare their clothing, while the older men and

Figure 6.2 Members of the Young Men's Association
carry the *mikoshi*

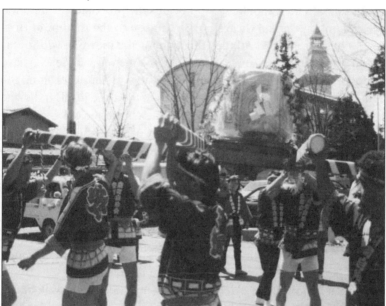

the vice-head of the Young Men's Association sit in a circle on the floor and confirm the route for the processional and what needs to be done along the way, including specific rest areas and points at which the truck carrying the children will stop to perform. All of the men involved with this meeting have performed *kabōsai* many times in their lives and are completely aware of how the procession operates. Thus, the actual consultation seems less significant than the importance of the meeting as formal confirmation of the advisory role of the elder men as they instruct the vice-head of the Young Men's Association on the day's events.

When the meeting ends, women bring cups of saké and the elder men raise their glasses to toast the beginning of the festival. A few minutes later, members of the Young Men's Association who will carry the *mikoshi* get up from the portion of the floor on which they have been sitting—an area that is separated from that of the elder men—and offer a toast of their own. At about 8:30am, the group of young men walks to the location where the *mikoshi* has been setup, lifts it up onto their shoulders, and begins the procession around the town shouting *wasshoi* (heave ho!) in unison to the rhythm of trotting. The procession continues throughout the morning with occasional stops to rest, eat, and drink beer along the way. Those who have participated in the festival in prior years know which stores along the route will have particularly good offerings of food and drink and make sure to stop at these places. In 1996, one newspaper delivery company had the doors open displaying a wide array of snacks and beer for the hard-working men carrying the *mikoshi*, and as we ate and drank many of the men commented on how this particular store was always the best place to stop. At the rest stops, children abroad the truck carrying the drum players from the Children's Association perform, and at the end of each performance, members of the Young Men's Association throw rice cakes (*mochi*) into the crowd of children and elderly women. This invariably initiates a scramble and shoving match among young and old alike to see who can collect the most.

The most prominent elder men in the neighborhood walk ahead of the *mikoshi*. And just behind the *mikoshi*, several other elder men pull a wagon into which shop-keepers and householders drop money or small bags of rice as the *mikoshi* passes their shops (which are also usually their homes). The money and rice represent offerings to the *kami* being carried around in the *mikoshi*. As they receive the offerings, the men hand out paper good luck charms for fire safety. By noon, the procession is over and everyone gathers back at the meeting house. Among the first orders of business is counting the money received. The counting is divided among several men who are members of the Old Persons Club and a few in their fifties who work with money at their jobs. Younger men are excluded form the counting. After the counting is completed, it is then confirmed by one of the most prominent elder men in the neighborhood, a man who has held local political office in the Town Assembly and who is regarded as one of two or three central figures among the neighborhood headmen. In 1996, the total collected was ¥445,100 or about $4,450 at that time. Some of the money is divided among the age grade associations (discussed below) to be used for expenses related to the festival. Approximately one-third of the money is used for a post-festival party (*hanseikai*) for the adults and to buy sweets and presents for the children from the Children's Association.

The post festival party commences at 4:30 in the afternoon and continues into the late hours of the evening. It begins with congratulatory speeches and toasts and thanks for everyone's participation by the neighborhood headmen, who sit at a head table in an honored position in the front of the room. The types of age-based segregation observed prior to the festival, in which the young men and elder men interact only on a formal basis, continue in the context of the party. The members of the Young Men's Association and the Old Persons Club generally sit at separate tables. The head and vice-head of the Young Men's Association honor the headmen by pouring them beer, saké, or other drinks. The elders reciprocate by pouring drinks for the younger men who worked hard to carry the *mikoshi*. This follows Japanese patterns of etiquette in which persons of lower status pour for persons of higher status, which may then be reciprocated by the person of higher status (Befu 1993:132). The pouring of drinks (particularly alcohol) in Japan carries symbolic meaning in that it indicates that the one pouring is at the service of the recipient (Befu 1993:130). The age-based power structure of the neighborhood continues to be expressed via the interactions among participants in the party, although it does become more relaxed as the party progresses and people become increasingly drunk.

Age and the Structure of Kabōsai

As with the practice of *omairi* discussed in the previous two chapters, age is an important variable in determining who participates and the particular capacity in which they are involved in *kabōsai*. However, unlike *omairi*, in which age is an informal determinant of participation and the age-based divisions of involvement are vaguely defined, in the *kabōsai* festival age is structurally built into the administration and performance of the ritual, with clear divisions of work and participation based upon membership in specific age-based associations of town folk. In order to understand the importance of age, and particularly of elders, in the administrative and participatory structures of the festival, it is necessary to go into some detail about the manner in which *kabōsai* is organized and run.

The administrative structure of *kabōsai* is built around age grading practices that are widely evident in the social organization of agricultural areas of Japan, but which can also be found in various forms in urban centers (Hendry 1981; Norbeck 1953; Traphagan 1998c, 2000a). *Kabōsai* is administered at the level of neighborhood self-government associations (*jichikai*). These associations consist of a variety of departments (*bu*) including several age-stratified associations that resemble the age grade patterns of social organization described by Evans-Pritchard in relation to East Africa (Evans-Pritchard 1940).[3] Throughout Kanegasaki and its surrounding areas, there are typically at least four age grade associations connected to the self-government associations that stratify communities into broadly defined groupings of age peers. These are the Old Persons Club[4] (*rōjin kurabu*), which includes people over the age of sixty; the Young Men's Association (*seinenbu* or *seinenkai*), which includes men from entrance into the workforce until age 42 (*yakudoshi*) or older in some cases; the Women's Association (*fujinbu* or *fujinkai*), which includes women from marriage or childbirth until entrance into the Old Persons Club; and the Children's Association (*kodomokai*), which includes students in grades one through six (Traphagan 1998c, 2000a). Membership in each association is based upon a combination of age in calendar years, as well as ascribed and adopted age-identities that categorize people as belonging to a particular period in the lifecourse, such as middle age, childhood, or old age. In each association, there is normally a strong cohort affiliation among the members, particularly among women as they move from the *fujinbu* (or *fujinkai*) to the *rōjin kurabu*.

In the past, age grade associations like these—particularly the *fujinkai* and *seinenkai*—were closely connected to nationalist movements supporting Japanese imperialism during the late 19th and early 20th Centuries. Women's associations, for example, were used by the national government to drum up nationalistic fervor and to support war efforts, such as in the Russo-Japanese War (Tamanoi 1998:48–49). And the *seinenkai*, using the term, *seinen*, which literally translates as "youth" and conveys, as Mariko Tamanoi notes, a sense of gender equality, was a framework through which the state could employ the concept of "equality to mobilize everyone, irrespective of gender, class, and even race for Japan's imperial expansion" (1998:51). In contemporary rural society, local chapters of the national *seinenkai* and *fujinkai* continue to operate, along side the neighborhood versions known as *seinenbu* and *fujinbu*, although in Kanegasaki these are not connected with each other. And while the *seinenkai* in Kanegasaki involves both men and women, the neighborhood *seinenbu* are restricted in membership to men. While the promulgation of nationalist ideology no longer is central to these age grade associations, they continue to have at least marginal links to local and national governments, from which they receive some financial support.[5]

Indeed, the quasi-governmental aspect of age grade associations can be seen at the neighborhood or hamlet level in the fact that they are typically considered to be departments within the Self-Government Associations for each neighborhood. In Jōnai, for example, the Self-Government Association is broken into several departments, which include a general affairs department, education and physical education departments, a welfare department, and the age grade associations. These positions represent the different subdivisions of the Self-Government Association and the number of people who hold leadership positions in each.

In general, the age grade associations have specific work responsibilities in their respective neighborhoods and these responsibilities are to some extent managed by the Self-Government Association leadership. For example, in Jōnai the Children's Association is responsible for cleaning gutters along the sides of roads and collecting bottles and newspaper for recycling, the proceeds from which are used for group outings such as camping or ski trips. In Minamimachi, the *seinenbu* is responsible for managing that neighborhood's involvement in the *kabōsai* festival, under the supervision of the elders who are in charge of the Self-Government Association. Members of the *seinenbu* carry the *mikoshi* throughout the downtown area, and the association's director is also in charge of all organizational aspects of the festival related to Minamimachi (again, under the supervision of neighborhood elders). Finally, the Woman's Association organizes fire awareness walks around the neighborhood, in which every house is visited to discuss fire prevention, and prepares food and drink for a variety of neighborhood gatherings and meetings.

Interestingly, in contrast to the other age grade associations, in general the Old Persons Clubs lack formally assigned work responsibilities in the neighborhoods in Kanegasaki, although in Mizusawa I have encountered one neighborhood in which the Old Persons Club is responsible for park beautification. Nevertheless, virtually all positions of political leadership in the community are held by male members of the Old Persons Club, exceptions being the head of the Children's Association, the Mother's Traffic Safety group, and in several cases those departments associated with health and welfare. It should be noted that it is not uncommon for the head of the Woman's Association to be a prominent older man, even when the daily operation of the group is carried out by its female members, who consult with the male leader when needed. The centrality of elder men in the power structure of the community is quite evident in the power structure of the *kabōsai* festival. In all cases in the festival, leadership or advisory positions are held by men in their mid-sixties to late-seventies who are members of the Old Persons Club.

This situation is by no means unique to the *kabōsai* festival in Kanegasaki. For example, one of the largest festivals in the Tōhoku region, Akita City's *Kanto matsuri*, exhibits age stratification in leadership similar to that of *kabōsai*. *Kanto matsuri* dates back to the 18th Century and attracts more than ten thousand people to the four-day event held annually in August. Seventy teams with a total of nearly 1000 people of all ages participate as performers and musicians, the central attraction being the use of long bamboo poles on which paper lanterns are hung.[6] These poles weigh more than 50kg each and are balanced by performers on the palms of their hands, shoulders, hips, and among the most skilled, their foreheads. The performances of each team are judged, thus the festival represents more than entertainment, being a competitive event among the teams involved. This festival is controlled by an executive committee (*jikko iinkai*) that has 32 members. The Mayor of Akita sits as committee chair and most members are over the age of 65 and have participated in the festival for as much as 40 years. Furthermore, elder members of the community who have performed in the festival are those responsible for acting as judges of the events.

Schnell points out that, for the festival he studied in Gifu Prefecture, there is a clearly defined hierarchical chain of command related to the performance of the festival. Orders are passed from the elders, who function as shrine representatives, to the director of the festival and on down through the group dealing with the *yatai* (a wheeled float) and then to the neighborhood, household, and specific families involved (Schnell 1999:118–19). This system is used for passing information and assigning quotas of personnel who will be involved in carrying out the activities involved with the festival (Schnell 1999:118). The importance of elder men in this hierarchy, whether in Gifu, Akita, or Kanegasaki, revolves around their position as formal and informal leaders in the community. Although membership in the Old Persons Club is not mandatory, men who do not belong rarely hold positions of power or influence in neighborhood politics. In Kanegasaki, responsibility for running *kabōsai* rotates each year among the neighborhoods that make up the downtown area. The individual who heads the Self-Government Association for a particular neighborhood becomes the director of the festival for the year it is allocated to his neighborhood and he is appointed director of the festival committee, which meets annually, about a month prior to the date of the festival. Twenty men, all of whom hold leadership positions in their respective neighborhoods and all of whom are in their late sixties and seventies, form the committee along with the eleven representatives (*sōdai*) to Kanegasaki Shrine, which is the focal point of the festival. Others attend the meeting, including the head of the local association of businesses (*shōkōkai*), which plays a major role in the festival.

Aspects of celebration in *kabōsai* reflect what Grimes refers to as "expressive play" (1982:48). This is evident in the traditional costumes worn by riders on the *yatai* and carriers of the *mikoshi* and in the clown suits worn by the 25-year-old *yakudoshi*. To be sure, the procession is a form of entertainment in which people enjoy wearing both elaborate and humorous costumes and partake of drinking and food as they move about the town. In the past this was one of the primary elements of the festival throughout the entire town; some of the older townspeople described it as one of the few forms of entertainment available when they were young, prior to the time of television, movies, and *pachinko*[7] parlors. People would gather for *kabōsai* and the few other festivals that occurred throughout the year to enjoy a break from the labors of farming and to be distracted from the poverty that many experienced. Today much of the entertainment value of the festival is directed at children. Along with the procession, one of the main streets is lined with booths for purchasing various kinds of festival foods such as fried noodles (*yakisoba*) and corn dogs. There are also games available for children to play and several booths set up at which adults can purchase beer.

To understand the relationship between the ritual performance and the elderly, however, the most useful theoretical framework is one that focuses upon the social structural function of the ritual as it unfolds within the fabric of meaning that endows elders with symbolic capital on the basis of having attained old age, and that reinforces their position in the community as managing collective concern through the festival ceremony (Geertz 1973:146). Akiko Hashimoto makes the important point that in Japan the elderly are differentiated as a group on the basis of their ascriptive status as elders. As such, they are a class of people who can legitimately expect care and protection from others, and social policies directed toward the elderly embrace and reflect these ideas about old age (Hashimoto 1996:40–43). This ascriptive status can be understood in terms of symbolic capital, or the ability to direct others toward specific ends based upon one's social position rather than on accrued prestige and power tied to individual accomplishments (social capital). Symbolic capital forms a kind of institutionally organized and, to some extent, guaranteed source of recognition (prestige) that incorporates power as an inherent feature of one's social position (Bourdieu 1977:171). Not only does ascriptive status as an elder legitimize certain frames of behavior in which one can depend upon others, it also brings with it the ability to, and expectation that one will, be involved in directing other, younger, members of the community. The attainment of elder status, which is structurally identified in agricultural areas like Kanegasaki in terms of having entered the elder age grade association, brings with it, particularly for men, a social position inherently endowed with symbolic capital. The context of public rituals such as *kabōsai* form public representations of elder men as religious leaders—leaders in the expression of collective concern.

It should not be assumed that simply being old is sufficient to become a neighborhood headman and leader of ritual performances such as *kabōsai*. Both gender and personal qualifications such as family status and wealth, prior experience in leadership positions, and accomplishment over a lifetime contribute to one's position within the elder age grade. However, having become a member of the Old Persons Club, and thus having attained elder status, automatically endows one with some degree of symbolic capital, thus making one eligible for these positions. The capacity to use symbolic capital associated with elder status is, in a sense, intensified for specific men who have also accrued social capital over their lifetimes as a result of personal accomplishments, such as the attainment of wealth, specific types of experience, or political power. And, indeed, exercise of a combination of social and symbolic capital characterizes the nature of elder male participation in *kabōsai*.

In large part, the role of the elder men consists of being advisors to the younger men who do most of the organizational work for the festival. Elder men attend organizational meetings in which work responsibilities are doled out and decisions are made about specific aspects of the festival in order to be available for advising if the need arises. For example, at one organizational meeting, a question arose about the route that the procession should follow. A new road had been built in the center of town and the planners were not sure if the procession should pass along this new road. The head of the Young Men's Association consulted with one of the elder men in the room, who, in turn, consulted with a small group of other elder men, and the decision was made not to lead the procession along this road. In this case, power for final decision-making rested with the elders.

It seems reasonable to argue that the power of the elder men is based on a combination of two traits that they hold. First, the simple fact of being elder men places them in a position of being final arbiters for decisions about the festival. This aspect of their power draws from symbolic capital—being old (and male) inherently endows one with some degree of decision-making power. But this alone is not enough, because these men also have accumulated knowledge (social capital) over years of involvement with the festival. This attribute—the cognitive memory or cultural knowledge which comes with growing older—is embodied in the elder men who are involved in the festival. In other words, the elder men are resources of cultural knowledge that is necessary for the festival to be run in a manner consistent with past festivals.

The position of elder men as holders of symbolic and social capital is recognized both in the deference of the younger men to their elders in decision-making, as well as in formal contexts in which the status of the elder men can be displayed. At meetings, and particularly at the post-festival party, the elder men are seated in honored positions at the head table in the room, and during the procession they take honored places at the front.

One way to interpret the performance of the context of the festival is as demonstrating, and thus legitimizing, through the presentation of religious symbolism, the power structures operating in the neighborhoods that participate in the ritual (Bloch 1989:208; Schnell 1995:309). The process of preparation and performance of *kabōsai* represents the ritualization of vertical oppositions of superior and inferior that are based on the opposition of elder and other (Bell 1992:125), a form of secular social stratification based upon sensitivity to rank order that is a central feature of Japanese social organization. More specifically in the case of *kabōsai*, the procession visually acknowledges the ascriptive status of elders as holders of symbolic capital derived from their age and membership in the elder age grade and legitimizes a gerontocratic form of social organization in which elder men are placed at the center of maintaining communal concern. The placement of elder men at the head of the procession and in honored positions during other aspects of the festival is central in the visual expression of social structure. I have observed older men who have, out of humbleness (a trait valued in Japanese society), chosen to walk toward the back of a procession, only to be brought to the front in order to take their appropriate position. The fact that the ritual is administered and organized in terms of the age grades reinforces the age grading practices that structure the life course and endow elder status with symbolic capital.

The performance of *kabōsai* represents a confined public expression of the age hierarchies operating in the neighborhoods. In short, the ritual encapsulates the entire social structure of the neighborhoods by itself being structured in terms of that structure. The ritual serves to synthesize and display the general ideas about social order that obtain in the neighborhoods (Geertz 1973:89); participation in the ritual and tacit acceptance of the position of the elders as advisors and leaders legitimizes or authorizes the culturally constructed hierarchies through which people organize political power (Kawano 1996:83).[8]

Concern and Kabōsai

The advisory role of the elders in the administrative structure of *kabōsai* is an example of the importance of the elderly in managing the expression of concern through ritual performance. But how is *kabōsai* an expression of concern and, more specifically, a representation of collective concern about the well-being of the members of the community? If we return briefly to the ethnographic vignette I presented to begin chapter one, collective concern was expressed in the purification of the elder men of the community at a New Year's Day ceremony. The men, and by extension the entire community they represent, receive the purification rites through which people are able to express their broad concern with communal well-being. In the speeches that open the ceremony, elder men rise to express general comments about the well-being of the community. The head of the *rengōkai* (Unity Association) does this explicitly by contrasting the positive year that Kanegasaki has experienced with the difficult times that seem to permeate Japanese society. The issue of concern about the well-being of the community is contextualized within the framework of the ritual actions that purify the elders who lead the community. In other words, the power, be it figurative or actual, of the *kami* is employed as a way of both purifying the leaders and expressing the concern of the residents over the well-being of the community in which they live.

Like the New Year ceremony, *kabōsai* also accomplishes this in an even broader manner by taking the *kami* within the *mikoshi* around the neighborhoods, thus ritually purifying the entire community. During the meetings for preparation of the festival, in addition to members of the Young Men's Association, the one other group of younger people who are involved are those at an age in life known as *yakudoshi*. This term indicates particular years in the lifecourse in which one is likely to experience misfortune. The specific years that are marked in this way are ages 1, 4, 7, 10, 13, 16, 19, 23, 25, 28, 33, 40, 42, 46, 49, 51, 55, 58, and 61 (Brown 1979:221). Men at age 42 and women at age 33 are viewed as being particularly vulnerable because they are in the *yakudoshi* year known as *taiyaku*, which literally means "big calamity" indicating that these ages have the highest potential for disaster among all of the inauspicious years. In relation to the performance of *kabōsai*, those who are in *yakudoshi* years represent "liminal *personae*," people in need of ritualized assistance as they make the transition through a period in life that is perceived as being particularly dangerous (Turner 1977:95). *Kabōsai* provides a context in which special ritual attention—the expression of concern—can be given by placing those in *yakudoshi* into close proximity to the *kami* in a way that is beyond the usual activities of going to a shrine to request particular benefits through *omairi*.[9]

It should be pointed out that even with this public ritual expression of concern about those who are in *yakudoshi*, it is common for those who are about to enter *yakudoshi* to make a concerted effort to visit a shrine at the New Year in the year they turn 33 or 42, and there are also special ceremonies for *yakudoshi* in which one can participate with others in the same situation at many shrines. Although many in *yakudoshi* who participate in these rituals do so for purposes of entertainment or for practical reasons such as the possibility of meeting new people (particularly those of the opposite sex for the unmarried), the importance of the *yakudoshi* in the festival can certainly be interpreted as one example of the expression of concern. There is an underlying sense among some that participation in the ritual functions to counteract potential dangers of being at one of these ages. However, attitudes about the actual power of the *kami* and the importance of performing rituals associated with *yakudoshi* are often ambivalent. As one woman, Yamamoto Yukiko, stated:

> I did do *yakuburai* [ritual purification for *yakudoshi*] at the shrine on New Year of my 33rd year. I received *omamori* and [a representation of] *fudo* [a Buddhist deity often called upon to protect against calamity or disaster] that I kept for the entire year, then at the next New Year I went back to the shrine and returned these to be burned. I did this primarily because people around me told me I should do this. I'm not all that sure why. I guess I did it because I was in *yakudoshi* and that's what you do when you are in *yakudoshi*.

Yamamoto's analysis of her involvement in shrine rituals associated with *yakudoshi* underscores her ambivalence about participation. On the one hand, she followed the rituals as expected. However, her purpose in doing this rested in the idea that it is simply what is done and what she was told to do, rather than any commitment to the idea that the rituals or the *kami* associated with them had any power to influence the outcome of the dangerous year. Indeed, the fact that others were concerned about her well-being, indicated by their encouragement of her participation in the ritual, is reciprocated in her willingness to be involved with little reflection on the actual power of the rituals to protect her. For some, participation in *kami*-related rituals also often has a precautionary aspect to it—one should at least take appropriate precautions in the event that *yakudoshi* is truly a potential hazard in life (Reader and Tanabe 1998:62–63). In other words, it is better to avoid taking any chances and do the ritual, just in case the powers of the deities are real.

While those in *yakudoshi* are an important focus for the expression of collective concern in *kabōsai*, other elements of the festival, such as the *mikoshi* and *yatai*, also represent frames through which concern is expressed. As noted above, the *yatai* is a large, wheeled float on which ride several young girls who are dressed in kimono and have their faces covered in white make-up with rouge on their cheeks and their hair done up with flowers. In the past, the *yatai* carried 19-year-old women (who were in *yakudoshi*), and who were considered eligible wives. One of the organizers of the event, who had participated in the festival since its early days, noted that the *yatai* was a way to circulate the women in beautiful costume about the town, displaying them as potential brides for the single men. However, in recent years, due to a shortage of women the appropriate age, the focus of the *yatai* on marriage-aged women has not been possible and now the *yatai* includes girls in middle school who have learned to play the *shamisen,* and elementary school girls (1st through 3rd grades) who have learned to play Japanese drums (*taiko*). And, of course, the *mikoshi,* by its very nature in bringing the *kami* out of the main shrine to purify the entire area indicates an expression of collective concern for the well-being of the community. In other words, concern and the importance of elder men in managing the expression of concern are via *kabōsai* represented publicly through the structure and performance of the ritual.

Gender, Age, and Domains of Ritual Practice

In the above description, I have devoted considerable attention to the political importance of elder men in the community, and the representation of their status through the public ritual of *kabōsai* because the pattern evident closely follows tendencies in Japanese society to structure gender roles around inner and outer spheres of activity. Dorinne Kondo argues that ideologies associated with the domestic sphere, including those supported by the state, "define women in the interwar and postwar periods through their association with *uchi* [inside], the domestic domain" (1990:280). This role is associated with concepts of nurturance and devotion to the betterment of her family, and, as Vogel argues, is comparable to the singular devotion to work that is often attributed to the corporate worker (Vogel 1963, Kondo 1990:281). This singular devotion to work is part of the *soto* (outside) domain to which men, particularly those in white-collar professions, are viewed as devoting their lives. These two domains are represented as being separate "professional" spheres in which women carry out the responsibilities of the domestic sphere, nurturing and caring for the members of their households, and men carry out the responsibilities of the public sphere—devoting themselves to work, community, politics, and so on—in essence, nurturing the development of the public realm.

While this division of gender roles into domestic and public spheres is important in Japanese society, it is necessary to avoid overstating the division. Women can and do devote themselves to the public sphere. They run for political office (and sometimes win) and they have careers and focus their lives on the company, although many women who stay in the working world for a career remain single, marriage being a basis on which to leave work and focus attention on the *uchi* domain (cf. Ogasawara 1998). And in some cases, men choose to stay home and raise the children, although this is rare. Nonetheless, the sharp, gendered division of domains of activity is an important and broadly evident part of Japanese life.

In this and the previous two chapters, I have shown that the connection between gender and these domains extends to the realm of ritual performance. Elder men are largely responsible for managing the rituals of the public sphere—the rituals of the festivals and ceremonies that are devoted to communal, public well-being. Men are the "priests" of public ritual activities—indeed, not only are elder men in lay leadership roles, but priests (whether Buddhist or Shintō) are invariably men. While keeping in mind the limitations of the metaphor, it is reasonable to argue that elder women, by contrast, are, as Lebra (1984:289) suggests, the "priestesses" of the household, managing the domestic sphere of ritual performance. In short, the role of lay religious leader in Japan is structured around both age and gender. The elderly are the ones primarily responsible for carrying out ritual performances, and the spheres of these performances are divided along gendered lines of public and domestic roles as is common throughout Japanese society.

What is interesting about this gendered division of labor is less the fact that it is divided, but the fact of how it is divided. Both elder men and women carry out the same basic types of tasks as ritual leaders. In short, both men and women take leadership roles in terms of the expression of concern through ritual performance. The difference lies less in the role itself than it does in the domain of activity in which the role is enacted. It is the emphasis on concern that is central to understanding the relationship between the elderly, religious or ritual participation, and well-being in Japan. Elder men and women are the main performers in the lifelong care system that I have been discussing throughout this book. Their responsibilities vary in that the role of men is more focused on the public sphere of expressing concern and carrying out rituals that will maintain the well-being of the community; the role of women is more focused on the domestic sphere in which concern about the well-being of one's family members is at the center of ritual attention. These are not, however, exclusive areas of behavior. Women do sometimes become involved in leadership roles in rituals such as *kabōsai*, although this is quite rare. And men can involve themselves in domestic rituals, or rituals at shrines and temples, at any time and to the extent that they wish. What should be clear at this point is that both elder men and women involve themselves as nurturers in the context of ritual performance. Elder men carry out the responsibilities of nurturing the well-being of the public sphere; elder women carry out the responsibilities of nurturing the well-being of the domestic sphere.

Chapter 7

Old Age, Ritual, and Concern

At the temple visitor's lodge
My sick friend appears dancing in a dream,
When I awake
Rain strikes the stones beneath the temple eaves.[1]

—Itoh Setsuko

In January of 1999, the U.S.-based John E. Fetzer Institute issued a publication entitled *Multidimensional Measurement of Religiousness/Spirituality for use in Health Research*. The report makes the important point that variables connected to religious behavior or spirituality "cannot simply be combined into a single scale that examines the effects of a single variable, religiosity…" (1999:2). Developed by a working group that consisted of an interdisciplinary collection of scholars including sociologists, psychologists, and specialists in public health and medicine, the report identified various "domains of religiousness/spirituality" such as "meaning," "values," "beliefs," "forgiveness," "religious/spiritual coping," "commitment," and several other categories that affect health and that are in need of further research (1999:4). Identification of these domains, and other domains such as hope, compassion, or mystical experience, is an important element of the report and recognizes the limitations of simplistic treatments of religious and spiritual behavior as it relates to health and well-being. Following the introduction, the report includes sets of questions intended for use by researchers. These questions are organized in terms of the domains that the working group identified. There is a considerable breadth of topics covered in the domains. Examples include the importance of faith in one's life (values domain, page 28), the magnitude of "God's goodness and love" (belief domain, page 32), the importance of having children believe in "God" (belief domain, page 32), concerns about forgiveness and confession by others and by "God" (forgiveness domain, page 36), frequency of reading the Bible or other religious materials (private religious practices domain, page 38), the frequency of feeling "loved and cared for" by one's congregation (religious support domain, page 62), and frequency of involvement in religious services (religious/spiritual history domain, page 68). The goal of many of the questions associated with these domains is to provide a basis for finding statistical correlations between health (whether in terms of subjective reporting or objective measures such as blood pressure) and various domains of religious/spiritual activity and belief.

My purpose in citing this report is neither to challenge the usefulness or the validity of the domains identified, nor to question the instruments developed by the working group. Indeed, the report provides a very useful tool for considering religion and health in American Christian contexts. Rather, my aim is to point out the limitations of the approach, which become quite clear as one examines the culture-boundedness of the domains identified in the report and the difficulties in applying these domains in contexts such as Japan. Indeed, there have been attempts to draw conclusions from the study of religion and health in Japan using these types of domains (Krause et al. 2002; Krause and Ingersoll-Dayton 1999). However, these studies have been hampered by a tendency to frame Japanese religious activities within the Western conceptualization of religion *qua* "faith" rather than searching for an emic language of ideas related to religious performance. As the data I have presented here show, there are serious difficulties in applying the types of categories outlined in the Fetzer Institute report to the Japanese context of "religious" behavior—at least without significant modification. One's congregation in Japan does not usually provide a context for feeling loved and cared for in the sense normally associated with church congregations in the West, although ritual performance is clearly an expression of emotional attachment and concern with others. Frequency of involvement in religious services is simply not relevant for understanding much of Japanese religious behavior because most of that behavior is situational or allocated to specific members of a household. Participation depends upon situation, such as the need to express concern about a sick relative or friend, or the arrival at a particular lifecourse transition such as marriage, or may be conducted by a particular individual on behalf of the entire household. Questions related to the magnitude of "God's" love, forgiveness, kindness, and so on are completely irrelevant in the Japanese context—the deities, to the extent that people are even concerned with them, behave as humans, showing kindness, hatred, evil, and good. The assumption that a spiritual agent such as "God" is associated with love, forgiveness, or kindness is a Christo-centric perspective that simply does not apply in contexts such as Japan. While concerns about healing, health, and well-being are clearly central in Japanese religious practice, these are generally not framed in terms of faith, even though there may be practical benefits associated with participation in ritual performance.

While Japan is a particularly good example of a non-faith and non-belief centered approach to religious practice, it is by no means unique. The notion that doctrine and theology are central to religious practice is of limited applicability elsewhere in Asia. As Flood notes in relation to Hinduism,

> [r]itual...cuts across theological distinctions. If it is possible to define Hinduism, it is certainly not possible to do so in terms of doctrine and theological beliefs. Ritual is prior to theology, both historically and conceptually, and various theologies in India have been built upon a ritual basis and make sense only in the context of ritual traditions (Flood 1996:199).

There are a variety of examples from Asia that one could cite in terms of the relative downplaying of doctrine and theology in comparison to ritual, as well as a tendency towards syncretism in relation to sectarian affiliation and practice, however these tendencies are found in other parts of the world, as well. Frank Lipp notes that although the religion of the Mixe people in Oaxaca, Mexico is Roman Catholicism, "for a variety of historical reasons, the religion that has evolved is to some degree syncretic, embodying traditional pre-Hispanic beliefs and practices as well as those of European origin" (Lipp 1991:24). Lipp offers the interesting observation that this has generated a situation in which there is a symbolic system from which "each individual, to some extent, selects and emphasizes particular religious themes of the total symbolic complex" (Lipp 1991:24). This, as Lipp notes, tends to make cultural generalization difficult.

One can continue along this path, citing examples from numerous cultures in which religious practice is structured around a primacy of ritual, but the basic point is simple and clear; a key element in the domains that need to be identified—culture—has been left out of the Fetzer Report. It is instructive that at the end of the report there is a category for religious preference. This section of the report includes a list of four Jewish sects from which one can choose, a brief list of non-Western religions including Buddhism, Shintō, Hinduism, Islam, Taoism, and Baha'i, a category for Wiccan or other forms of "ritual magic,"[2] and 59 categories for Christian-oriented groups and sects (1999:84). As I have shown throughout this book, even the idea of having a "religious preference" makes little sense in the Japanese context, where one engages different institutional frameworks depending upon the particular ritual task—for example, a Shintō shrine or Christian church for a wedding or a Buddhist temple for a funeral. For the most part, Japanese simply do not organize their religious/ritual activities in terms of "preference," instead organizing these activities in terms of pragmatic goals and situations.[3] While there are some contexts in which the idea of religious preference makes sense, such as for the new religions like Sōka Gakkai or for Christian groups, Japanese generally do not engage in religious activity in this way. Even among individuals who belong to traditional sects such as Jōdō Shinshū—whose founder, Shinran (1173–1262), has been compared with the Protestant reformer Luther on the grounds that he conceptualized faith as a gift from Amida Buddha and emphasized the idea that "faith, or salvation is not due at all to the contriving action of man but [arises] solely through the power of Amida Buddha" (Bloom 1965: 45)—in practice exclusivity of "preference" or belonging is rarely found.

This lack of exclusionary sectarian affiliation is readily evident in the neighborhood of Jōnai in Kanegasaki, where virtually all of the residents belong to the parish (*danka*) of the local Soto Zen temple, largely due to the samurai heritage of many of the residents. Among this group there is a long tradition (at least 300 years) of carrying out the ritual of the *nembutsu*—the repeated chanting of the phrase *namu amida butsu* (also discussed in chapter 4), which within religious texts is represented as the means by which one can attain salvation or entrance into the Buddhist Pure Land (Bloom 1965:18). Members of the neighborhood gather on the evening of a funeral in the house of the deceased. The participants dress in the black clothing they wore for the funeral and sit in a circle in a large room in the house where a funeral altar has been erected. There they spend approximately twenty minutes chanting "*namu amida butsu*" while passing a large set of beads that encircles the room through their hands. When I asked participants to discuss this ritual, they did not frame it in terms of salvation. Rather, as one informant explained, "we do this to assist the deceased in his or her journey—wherever that may be." Perhaps the key phrase here was "wherever that may be" in that this points to the ambiguities that surround Japanese concepts of the afterlife. In another instance of discussing the afterlife, I asked a Buddhist priest where the ancestors are located. After asking the question several times, each time receiving a quizzical look from the priest, I asked if it was a stupid question. He responded to this with an emphatic "yes." From a theological perspective, this may well have been a stupid question, but, as noted in chapter 4, from the perspective of a lay person, this would have been reasonable. Many lay persons very much think in terms of actual place, such as the *butsudan*, *ihai*, (the tablet on which the deceased's posthumous name is written), or grave as the location of the ancestor (cf. R. Smith 1974; Keith Brown, personal communication). This underscores the general lack of interest in theological issue that characterizes much of the laity in Japan.

In fact, in reference to the performance of the *nembutsu* the lack of concern over the sectarian connection of the ritual was noted when it was explained that in the past the ritual was kept secret from the Zen priests, as were other *nembutsu*-related rituals (*kakushi nembutsu*) practiced by people living in the region. By contrast, in contemporary Jōnai, the time and place of the *nembutsu* are announced at the end of the funeral service held in the Zen temple.

Perhaps another approach to take in addressing this issue is to argue that Japanese people simply do not involve themselves in religious activity. What they do at shrines, temples, or at home is merely a matter of ritual. Japanese themselves often indicate that they are not "believers" in any particular god or set of gods, but they will not deny that they are practitioners of religiously framed forms of action. There is no necessary correlation between religious activity and belief in spiritual beings.

It is clear from the ethnographic data I have presented in this book that the fact that people participate in festivals, regular *omairi*, or visits to temples and shrines on an as-needed basis should not be construed as implying that they are necessarily "believers" in the deities or in the powers of the deities that are associated with the sacred spaces or ritual acts that they engage. One may find virtually any level of engagement ranging from notions that Buddhist and Shintō entities have some sort of power, to ambivalence, to outright lack of belief in the power or presence of these entities. But there remains a sense that it is customary to carry out activities like visiting a shrine at appropriate times, such as the beginning of one's *yakudoshi* year, and that shrine visitation and participating in religious ritual, if not invoking the power of the deities, at least serves the purpose of refreshing or cleansing oneself psychologically or spiritually. This point was raised by several informants in relation to both ancestor-oriented and *kami*-oriented rituals. Several informants indicated that daily practice of ancestor rituals brings a sense of "serenity" (*otonashii*) to one's inner self (*kokoro*), as noted previously. The practical, calming, and often cleansing or purifying aspects of participation in these ritual activities was summed up well by Kawamura Yoshiko, who was about to turn 33 at the time we spoke. When I asked her why she was participating in shrine-related *yakudoshi* events (mentioned in the previous chapter, as well), she explained her participation in the following way:

JWT: Do you believe in the *kami*?

Kawamura: I don't believe in the *kami*, but I will go to the shrine to participate in the shrine festival tomorrow.

JWT: When you go, will you do *oharai*? [This is a form of purification done by the priest that was discussed at the beginning of chapter 1.]

Kawamura: Yes. And I did it at the New Year this year because of *yakudoshi*. It isn't that I don't believe in the *kami* 100 percent, I guess I believe in *kami* about 10 percent.

JWT: Then, if you 90 percent do not believe in *kami*, why do you do rituals related to them?

Kawamura: It's custom. I did it at this year's New Year. There is a ceremony called *yakubarai* done at the shrine. This is to cleanse people who are entering into *yakudoshi*. I don't really know why we do this ritual. Maybe sometime in the past a lot of women died around the age of 33. At that time the normal life span was only until about 50 years old. So at 33, half of one's life was over.

JWT: Why did you do rituals related to *yakudoshi* if you 90 percent don't believe in this sort of thing?

Kawamura: Well, do you understand the meaning of *oboreru* [to be drowned]? I felt like I was drowning (in life) and I thought that by doing the ritual it might help to wipe away the negative environment that was surrounding my life. For example, at times when I thought that I very badly wanted to get married I would have really bad feelings. I felt depressed. I wanted to remove the bad environment and have a new start to my life. I wanted to wash off all of the negative things and start a new life.

JWT: So that's why you did the ritual for *yakudoshi*?

Kawamura: Yes.

JWT: Was there any other reason?

Kawamura: No. Well, afterwards there is a party. And that is an opportunity to meet new people. Women dress up in kimono. Because there aren't many parties like that in Japan, I thought that it was a chance. Entering their 33rd year, women go to the shrine for the ritual. It's done as a group thing and there is a party afterwards at which there are also men. So there is an opportunity to meet men there. The men are not at the ritual, but they go to the party. However, by this age, virtually all of the men are married. So that was one of my purposes in going. There is also an opportunity to meet some old friends who I hadn't seen for many years and it was a bit of a nostalgic feeling.

Within the span of two sentences, Kawamura moves from stating clear disbelief in the *kami* to a degree, small as it is, of ambivalence about their existence and their powers. Undoubtedly this is at least partially, and I suspect largely, a result of my own influence by asking the question in the way I did, using the term *shinjiru* (to believe) in reference to the *kami*. This term is not one that people necessarily associate with religious practice or with the *kami*, but, instead, was developed in the 19th Century as a scholarly term to be used in writing about Christianity (Reader and Tanabe 1998). Her initial answer to why she does the rituals—that it is custom—is typical of what many Japanese state as a reason for their involvement in religious rituals. But what is "custom" in this context? I think it reasonable to argue that carrying out these rituals is a customary way of expressing concern. Kawamura uses the ritual associated with *yakudoshi* to put into action her concerns about her own marital status and the "negative environment" that she indicates was permeating her life. The renewal that she hopes to gain from her actions is commonly associated with Shintō ritual practice at the New Year in particular, but also at other times, and, as Nelson (1996:199) notes, "[i]t takes a considerable amount of ill luck and cynicism before an individual in Japan will regard the ending of the old year and the beginning of the new as being without hope and fresh possibilities."

Through her hope for cleansing and renewal via the *yakudoshi*-related practices, Kawamura is enlisting the therapeutic aid, not of the *kami*, but of the ritual and ceremony that surrounds the New Year and her specific categorization as *yakudoshi*. This is an expression of her concern over her own psychological well-being and, perhaps, because she had been pressured about marriage by family members, concern about the well-being of her relatives (particularly her parents). In other conversations, Kawamura explained that she encountered constant "nagging" from relatives about her need to marry, an experience that is common for unmarried women in their thirties and unmarried male or female successor children like Kawamura in particular (see Traphagan 2000a, 2004). She explained that she thought it would be useful from both psychological and practical perspectives to participate in the ritual as a way of dealing with this pressure. While cleansing her inner self, she might even have the opportunity to meet an eligible male.

Belief is at best peripheral to her involvement in the shrine rituals. If we interpret Kawamura's behavior as ultimately not religious on the basis that it is not based on belief in spiritual agencies, we would end up sidestepping the issues of both meaning and agency that are central to her engagement of sacred spaces and religiously oriented ritual activity. Rather than concerning ourselves with belief, it may be more productive to return to the issue of concern, specifically Tillich's emphasis on the notion of ultimate concern with being.

Within modern Western thought, the idea that belief is central to religious life has become so natural that we rarely question or consider the meaning of the word and its historical development in relation to religion and other domains of human activity. Indeed, I think it is reasonable to argue that the association of belief with religion in Western societies can be understood in terms of Bourdieu's notion of the *doxic* mode, which I view as a domain of experience in which subjective principles of organization—whether epistemological, social, or behavioral—appear so natural that they are viewed as being objectively self-evident (Bourdieu 1977:164). Within this doxic mode, belief and knowledge are set apart as distinct domains in which belief represents subjectivity and knowledge objectivity. Knowledge, as Wittgenstein (1969:25e) notes so clearly in *On Certainty*, relies upon the assumption that what is known is grounded in some external principle that gives credence to our experience. Knowledge is closely associated with certainty in that by grounding understanding in an external frame of reference, we are able to remove doubt about the verity of what we know. Belief, by contrast, admits to the possibility of uncertainty—that there may be alternate ways of conceptualizing experience and understanding.

This juxtaposition of belief and knowledge, and through extension the association of religion with belief, is a distinctively Western way of looking at the world, but the close association of religion with belief is by no means a necessary way of conceptualizing religious experience. Indeed, Wilfred Cantwell Smith (1977: 39) notes that in the Qur'an, the concept of 'belief' does not occur, raising questions about the utility of the category of belief as a way of understanding religious behavior and ideas even among historically related religions such as Islam, Judaism, and Christianity.

If we are to extend the study of the intersection of religion, health, and aging into the realm of cross-cultural and comparative research, we need to redirect our intellectual gaze away from the belief-oriented and church-centered approach that has guided research to date, and instead look for emic perspectives on how religion, health, and aging are tied together—if they are at all. In stating this, I am resorting to a very old argument in anthropology, one that appears in the first book to look at the intersection of ritual and health, and one of the earliest ethnographies that can be viewed as a form of medical anthropology, E. E. Evans-Pritchard's *Witchcraft, Oracles, and Magic among the Azande.*[4] In challenging readers to abandon simple objectivist positions concerning the religious and medical practices of other cultures, Evans-Pritchard makes the point that "Zande belief in witchcraft in no way contradicts empirical knowledge of cause and effect" (1976[1937]:25). Indeed, he states that the idea that death may occur through natural causes and may occur through witchcraft are not mutually exclusive. He notes that the Azande do not simplistically attribute the *cause* of an event to witchcraft—an elephant charging, in one of his examples, is the cause of a man's death, although witchcraft may have instigated the elephant to charge (1976[1937]:24). The death of the man by a rushing elephant is as much an empirical fact for the Azande as it is for us. But in the example Evans-Pritchard cites, the Azande explain this particular harmful event in terms of the practice of witchcraft. In other words, the Azande sees the same *how* of events that we see, but his interpretation of the reasons behind the event are based upon a different set of assumptions, one in which witchcraft is an important force in explaining why things happen, and specifically why they happen to particular people.

While in the West, particularly within the world of the academic, we would look for a different explanation—the man annoyed the elephant, or just happened to be in the wrong place at the wrong time—this is simply a different approach to explaining the reasons behind an event. The point here is that the idea that these expectations (e.g. witchcraft or coincidence) are necessarily opposed and that they need to be separated analytically is a position that derives from Western notions about the domains of objectivity and subjectivity, belief and knowledge, and, by extension, science and religion.

That religion is necessarily concerned with beliefs and forms a basis of subjective response to the world, is, like the example Evans-Pritchard gives us from the Azande, an assumption drawn from the Western predilection for dividing subject and object, belief and knowledge. But this association of religion with belief is not one that holds across cultural frames of experience. In the Japanese case, rather than being belief-centered, religious activity is practice-centered. That is, it is centered around the ritual practice focused upon the expression of concern about well-being—physical, psychological, and social—for oneself, one's family (including one's ancestors and descendants), one's community, and even one's nation. Ultimately, the Japanese case forces us to challenge the utility of analytic categories such as "belief" and "faith" for the study of religion and health.

It is clear from the ethnographic examples I have presented throughout this book, that for Japanese there is a close connection between concepts and practices related to health, well-being, care, and ritual performance. As I have argued, Japanese religious behavior can be understood as functioning like an HMO—as long as one keeps in mind the limits of this analogy—in which people engage in both preventive and remedial activities that revolve around the expression of concern through ritual performance. In other words, Japanese religious ritual performance can be understood as a complimentary health care system that supplements or augments the biomedical health care system. This complementary health care system is one in which elders take on the role of medical practitioner through their positions of leadership in executing and managing ritual performances related to the expression of individual and collective concern. For women, this is centered in the domestic sphere and for men in the public sphere, but both male and female elders often take important roles in carrying out the rituals of concern.

By presenting religiously oriented ritual practice in Japan as a type of health and well-being management system, and by placing the elderly at the center of this system as the ones who take on a central role in carrying out the rituals associated with the expression of concern (although, the preceding show that this is by no means limited to the elderly), it is necessary to return to the issue of the manner in which health and well-being are culturally constructed in Japan. Are health and well-being matters of the absence of disease or, as Alter asks, "the presence— statistically speaking—of a discernible pattern of low-risk behavior?" (Alter 1999:S43). Certainly, Japanese employ the biomedical perspective in conceptualizing health in terms of the absence of disease, and the Japanese government exhibits a strong interest in encouraging behaviors that reduce the risk of conditions such as heart disease and cancer. However, as I argued in chapter 3, health and well-being in Japan are conceptualized in a way that extends well beyond the biomedical realm and should be understood as a form of embodied capital.

Health and well-being are conceptualized not only in terms of the individual, but also in terms of the collective unit in which one lives. Devoting one's efforts to the maintenance of individual, and through that, collective well-being is not merely a matter of personal preference, but takes on *moral* implications. This is encapsulated in the concept of *ikigai*, which indexes a conceptualization of well-being that emphasizes the direction of one's efforts towards practically, and symbolically, making a sincere effort to maintain physical and mental health and well-being. The ritual activities I have described in the previous chapters are one means by which people do this. The concept of *ikigai* is closely linked to the expression of concern. The mere fact of having an *ikigai* indexes that one is concerned; going to shrines and temples to do *omairi* also indexes concern.

The point that I want to make here is that the theological language of Western religions is inadequate to the task of understanding how health and religion are tied together in the Japanese context. Indeed, not only is the language of Western religions inadequate, the language of biomedicine also is inadequate to the task of understanding how health and well-being are conceptualzed in the Japanese context. (cf. Good 1994:23). For Japanese, health and well-being are not restricted to individuals. Japanese conceptualize well-being in terms of their own individual health and success, the health and success of their family members and of the family as a unit, and the health and success of the communities in which they live. The boundaries among individual, family, and community are not necessarily sharply drawn in the Japanese way of looking at the world. While I want to avoid the often-presented "groupist" characterization of Japanese, it is important to recognize that for many Japanese the individual is fully realized as a human being within the context of social interaction (Traphagan 2000a, Smith 1984, Plath 1980). Well-being and health are not simply matters of autonomous individuals, although this is clearly important, but are also characteristics of individuals and the groups in which they involve themselves. Neither the biomedical nor the religious languages that have typically been used to explore the relationship between religion, health, and aging are likely to yield significant insights into the ways in which these concepts intersect in the Japanese context.

As I have argued, the concept that brings religion, health, and aging together in Japan is concern. Much of Japanese religious behavior is about expressing the emotions one experiences as one goes through the normal disappointments and joys that accompany life, through the guise of ritual performance. While anyone can do many of the rituals whenever needed, it is the elderly who carry the role of ongoing caretakers of the expression of the emotive ties that bind people together into families and communities. Through the daily performance of *omairi*, elder women ritually express the feelings of love for the deceased, but also love and caring (concern) for the living members of their families through contemplating the well-being of the family in front of the ancestors. Through the management of the shrine festivals such as *kabōsai,* elder men generate a context through which participants and spectators can ritually express their concern for their neighbors and the broader community in which they live. In short, elders are the caretakers of well-being and it is through ritual performance that much of their caretaking activities are carried out. The expression of concern is not a matter of voicing beliefs *about* concern for others; instead, it is a matter of *doing* concern about others.

In chapter 3, I looked at the concept of embodiment as it relates to memory and argued that our bodies can be understood as collections of past events, ideas, and experiences that we recollect and reinterpret constantly. Borrowing from Connerton, I suggested that in performing stylized movements and behaviors, we represent externally an embodied or sedimented past that consists of experiences and the interpretation of those experiences. Ritual acts, as Rappaport argues, can be understood as "markers," or observable units whose patterning conveys information-bearing symbols that are related to an ensemble of units (Rappaport 1999:112, Miller 1965:64). This notion of ritual as "observable" is worth exploring in greater detail. Henry Margenau uses this term in his philosophical work on quantum physics in a way that I think is useful here. An "observable is a kind of abstract quality, assigned as a latent attribute to objects; it somehow fills itself with content at the instants of observation" (Margenau 1977 [1950]:175). In other words, observables are latencies that are reified through the act of observation. The observable becomes "possessed" as a property through the act of observing others that surround it and ascribe meaning (properties) to it (Margenau 1977[1950]:175). By analogy, this seems to be very similar to the workings of ritual action. Rituals are markers that symbolically convey information about embodied experience—the latent attributes of individual humans and the collectivities they form. Experience becomes reified through the performance of the ritual.

In the case of the ritual activities in Japan that I have discussed throughout this book, it is the latent property of concern that is reified through the enactment of ritual action. In other words, ritual action reenacts in bodily form emotive meanings associated with the well-being of oneself and one's friends, family, and community. Through the performance of ritual, people come to not only feel concern, but to possess it as an observable property of lived experience, not simply a latent property of the individuals who experience life. The practice of ritual performance in Japan is the practice of concern. And it is the elderly who are the ones central in the *observation* of the rituals through which concern is reified.

As I have moved through the chapters in this book, I have tried to link together concepts of aging, religion, and health in a way that is different from what has typically been done in the gerontological literature on this topic. By infusing culture into the analytic landscape here, I have tried to show that these concepts, and indeed they are concepts, must be analytically framed in a way that reflects specific uses within cultural context. To be sure, all human societies have some concept of aging, some concept of religion and a system of ritual performances that go with it, and some notion of health, but it is very difficult, and ultimately may not be particularly intellectually profitable, to generalize beyond this point. For Japanese, that which is religious is centered not on belief, but on ritual—on the doing of concern, rather than the believing in the powers of spiritual entities to respond to or evoke our emotions. Health, taken as an emic concept, while certainly overlapping significantly with biomedical conceptualizations of health as typically found in Western societies, also must be understood as a subset of well-being, which encompasses not only an individual, but the collectivity in which he or she lives and interacts. For the elderly, much of well-being is centered around the pursuit of an *ikigai* or a reason or purpose in life, which has the functional properties of potentially staving off cognitive and physical decline.

Finally, it is the elderly who play a central role, at least in rural areas such as Tōhoku, in maintaining, or caretaking, well-being. The ultimate concern for the Japanese elderly I have discussed here is well-being, and it is through the ritual actions I have described that they reify that concern and make it not only the property, but the embodied possession, of themselves and the groups to which they belong.

Endnotes

Chapter 1

1. This action, as Nelson notes (1996:254) is directed at removing the "defilements, impurities, illness, evil, misfortune, and other impediments hindering the renewal of life energy" emanating from the Shintō deities (*kami*).

2. I use the term ceremony here in much the way that Grimes does. Ceremony is a special mode of ritual in which there is an intentional aspect to the ritualization of practice. There is a sense in which the actions associated with ceremony are directed toward a larger cause or reality. Unlike Grimes, however, I do not associate this with concepts of righteous or joyous acts—neither of which are necessarily associated with ceremonial behavior in Japan (Grimes 1982:41–42).

3. There are younger people involved in shrine ceremonies, particularly the shrine maidens (*miko*), or young women who typically work in shrine offices selling amulets and other religious objects and have roles in some ceremonies in which they dance to entertain the deities (Nelson 1996:260).

4. As an aside, it is worth noting that contemplating the importance of culture has theoretical consequences for the manner in which we conduct gerontological research concerning religion, health, and aging. By considering the relationship between religion and aging as I will throughout this book, I am indirectly also raising questions about the nature of gerontological knowledge production, which I in-

terpret as a social practice organized around the quest for causally defined certainty directed largely toward controlling processes (whether
social, psychological, or physical) of human aging. The gerontological discourse is an expression of the predilection in Euroamerican cultures to seek what Richard Rorty describes, in his book *Philosophy
and the Mirror of Nature*, as "epistemic comfort" and is the result of
a culturally circumscribed preoccupation with foundations "to which
one might cling, frameworks beyond which one must not stray, objects which impose themselves, representations which cannot be gain-
said", and, I would add, causes which lack ambiguity (Rorty
1979:315). In other words, the gerontological discourse is a product
of the Cartesian legacy that knowledge, in order to refute the skepti-
cal gaze, must be grounded in certainty (Johnson 1987:xxvi).

Gerontologists, perhaps because the field of gerontology has been
organized around representations associated with biomedical epis-
temology, have been particularly prone, whether searching for behavioral determinants of Alzheimer's disease, the relationship between spirituality and mental health, or correlations between
religious participation and "successful" aging, to structure inquiry
around the quest for theoretical generalization and unambiguous answers to our questions about the aging process. Recently, there has
been a growing body of work directed toward the development of a
critical gerontology that focuses on situating the behaviors of older
people within the dynamics of the narratives that shape interpretations of the aging process (cf. Cohen 1998). Culture in this approach
moves from being one among several objective variables that are
(usually unproblematically) fit into a model that describes, and perhaps attempts to predict behaviors and outcomes of aging persons,
to an often ambiguous and always polysemous fabric of ideas and
experiences through which aging persons, younger persons, and, of
course, gerontologists interpret and represent those behaviors and
outcomes. Central to the infusion of culture into the gerontological
landscape is the importance of recognizing that gerontology is itself
a product of culture, generated and maintained through what Lyotard refers to as the pragmatics of science, in which language
games—in the form of denotative utterances aimed at finding be-

ginnings (causes)—form the foundation upon which the institutions of knowledge production are built (Lyotard 1984:65). Gerontology is largely practiced through the semantics of objectivism, which guides the flow and creation of gerontological knowledge. Through the objectivist worldview, knowledge is disembodied from the subjective processes of human minds, as well as the cultural contexts that those minds generate, and is shifted to the abstract, "rule-governed manipulation of connections among symbols" that constitutes rational scientific inquiry (Johnson 1987:xxiv). Meaning is displaced from the complexities and polysemy of human imagination and abstracted into a realm of symbolic units that can be isolated, compared, correlated, categorized, and conceptually framed. And reality itself is viewed as an objective "other" onto which symbolic forms (language) can be mapped in a context-independent way (Johnson 1987:x).

Although the objectivist project is squarely aimed at separating meaning from the subjective processes of imagination that characterize human thinking, it is itself a product of those processes. Objectivism is a particular kind of narrative—a set of assumptions—that guide the direction of scientific practice. By defining objectivism as a narrative (indeed, it is a metanarrative that forms a court of highest appeal), I am unequivocally placing the social scientific endeavor, and thus gerontology, into the realm of social practice in which truths are produced within discourses that cannot be divorced from culture. Gerontology is practiced within a (meta)narrative that, as I use the term, is to be understood as the framework of possible meanings that limit and stimulate discourse (Schrag 1997:19). Narrative can be likened to the fake book (the chords and melodies) from which jazz musicians continually improvise. The basic structure of the tune is presented on the page, but the jazz musician can diverge from that both in terms of the melody and in terms of the chord changes. However, move too far away from this guide, and the connection to the original tune is lost and the acceptability of the diversion is challenged. In many areas of social science, and particularly within the realm of gerontology, objectivism forms the sole guiding principle through which data are collected, organized, and analyzed.

In situating gerontology and gerontological knowledge production within the frame of culture and narrative, I am not arguing that results and findings of objectivist gerontological research lack validity. Indeed, objectivist gerontological research has greatly increased our understanding of both biological and social aspects of the aging process, particularly in reference to people in industrialized societies. The point I want to emphasize here is that the objectivist endeavor is but one approach to the generation of knowledge; it is one epistemic setting that consists of specific (cognitive) structures that generate knowledge and shape the manner in which knowledge is articulated and interpreted (Cetina 1999:8). Indeed, the notion that this approach is a particularly good, or even the best, way to generate knowledge is an assumption, grounded in the cultures that have been heavily influenced by post-Enlightenment understandings of the world, that specific kinds of results—e.g. predictability—are the primary aim of any form of "scientific" research. Concepts such as well-being, spirituality, illness, health, and aging are usually framed and interpreted by social scientists within this epistemic setting rather than within other epistemic settings—such as those related to morality or values of normalcy and abnormalcy—through which people engage in the practice of generating discourse. In short, no deep understanding of how religiously oriented behavior, concepts of health and well-being, and the biological and social processes of aging are related can come about if we rely solely on the discourse of objectivism. Indeed, an uncritical reliance upon this approach inherently leads to ethnocentric and essentialist conclusions about the purposes and meanings associated with religious activity in later life, because it starts from a focus on the etic categories of the researcher, often overshadowing the emic categories through which people interpret experience.

5. I use the term "concepts" here to make a point that, while they can be seen as objective variables, health, religion, and aging are also conceptual categories that are used to interpret experience and processes related to the life course. Age, in particular, is often taken as an *a priori* biological fact that is not open to interpretation, but while the concept of age is often informed by biology, it cannot be

reduced to the biological manifestations of growing older (Trapha-gan 2000a:9). This has been pointed out very clearly by Meyer Fortes, who notes that chronological age and the manner in which stages of maturation of an individual over the life course are not necessarily associated. While age may be used as a measure of one's time on earth, the biological changes that occur as one ages are not necessar-ily the basis on which stages of maturation are conceptualized (Fortes 1984:101).

. This underscores some of the problems that arise in understand-ing the intersection of religion and aging, or other issues related to human behavior, if one pursues an uncritical reliance upon the types of positivistic approaches that are common in gerontological research. Subjectivity leaks into even the most "scientific" of research orienta-tions. The simple decision that one epistemological frame—that of positivism—is preferable or superior to others in terms of explain-ing behavior is based upon a set of assumptions about the nature of knowledge production. In the North American context, at least, ex-change rests at the foundation of knowledge production; the end of producing scientific knowledge is use-value (Lyotard 1984:16). This is particularly evident in the case of gerontology where most research, including that focused on religious behavior, is aimed at finding ways to control social and biological processes of aging.

There is another sense in which subjectivity enters into the research picture related to religion and aging. This is found in the dissocia tion, through a pragmatics of science that emphasizes use-value as the primary goal of knowledge production, of the basic "variables" which interest many researchers from the contexts and discourses in which they are invented, interpreted, and contested. The problem here lies in the fact that concepts, and their associated behaviors, such as religion, well-being, spirituality, and health are, to paraphrase Ly-otard, value-laden elements in heteromorphous networks of people and ideas that are interwoven and circulate among the individuals who make up social collectivities (1984:65). Furthermore, within these networks people engage in discourse—the interpretation of narrative—through which they contest and engage the narratives that they use to interpret the aging process and the extensive scientific literature that is written about that process. It is my contention that no real understanding of the relationship between religion/spirituality, aging, and health/well-being can come about without understanding the inherently contingent nature of each of these cultural categories. The meanings of religion, spirituality, aging, health, and well-being are culturally constructed and, thus, under constant pressure of interpretation and reinterpretation. As narratives and rhetorics are contested through discourse, they continually undergo processes of invention, reinvention, and improvisation. The contingent nature of these concepts necessitates beginning by exploring and problematizing their uses and meanings. See Rorty (1989) for an interesting discussion of contingency.

6. The HOPE acronym refers to "H—sources of hope, strength, comfort, meaning, peace, love and connection; O—the role of organized religion for the patient; P—personal spirituality and practices; E—effects on medical care and end-of-life decisions" (Anandarajah and Hight 2001:81).

Chapter 2

1. It is interesting to note that elder suicide has become a significant enough concern to be viewed as a social problem that is reported and discussed in the Japanese media. In one case, the popular weekly news magazine *Shūkan Shincho* (6 June 2002) was advertised in newspapers with the title "Male Suicide Rate Seven Times Higher than Women!" Although the article used in the advertisement actually dealt with elder suicide rates in the United States— it was an interview with an American who has written on the subject—the sensational and misleading aspect of the advertisement and the magazine's table of contents is suggestive of the concern in Japan with elder suicide.

2. This trend toward increased elder suicide in rural parts of Japan is not limited to the Tōhoku region. Matsumoto Toshiaki has found that in another rural prefecture, Niigata, the suicide rate for people under the age of 59 follows national averages, while the suicide rate for people over that age is generally above national averages. While

suicide rates have fallen nationally since the 1960's the rate for Niigata has remained significantly higher than the national average for those over the age of 65; in 1961 the national rate was 60.4, while the Niigata rate was 96.7; by 1990 the numbers had dropped to 39.6 and 59.5, respectively, but the differential between urban and rural prefectures remained significant (Matsumoto 1995:126). Indeed, Matsumoto's findings indicate that suicide rates in Japan rise in proportion to the agedness of the population, as well as to the depopulation of the region. In the rural county of Higashikubiki in Niigata, where Matsumoto focused his research, during the years from 1974 until 1987, 159 suicide cases occurred, with a suicide rate of 155.75, which is stunning when compared to the rate for Niigata as a whole (65.6) or the national rate of 41.3 over the same time (Matsumoto 1995:575).

3. Source: Japan Statistical Yearbook, Statistics Bureau, Ministry of Public Management, Home Affairs, Posts and Telecommunications (http://www.stat.go.jp/english/data/nenkan/zuhyou/b0226000.xls).

4. Source: Japan Statistical Yearbook, Statistics Bureau, Ministry of Public Management, Home Affairs, Posts and Telecommunications (http://www.stat.go.jp/english/data/nenkan/zuhyou/b0228000.xls).

5. This case is also discussed in Traphagan 2003a, Case 3 and in Traphagan 2004.

Chapter 3

1. Somewhat different versions of this discussion of the concept of *ikigai* appear in Traphagan forthcoming a and b.

2. I have discussed this particular pamphlet elsewhere in relation to the conceptualization of disability in Japan. See Traphagan forthcoming a.

3. As Akiko Hashimoto (1996) points out, unlike most Western societies, in Japan the identification of the elderly as a class of persons in greater need and at greater risk of becoming a burden is a legitimate form of social differentiation.

Chapter 4

1. This is not intended to imply that this is a system in precisely the same sense that a health care system is a system. There are distinct differences, including the fact that there is no overarching bureaucracy in the system of religious practice and institutions in Japan. In other words, it is not unified structurally. I do, however, think that there is a sense in which this is a unified system in the minds of the people who practice the associated rituals.

2. I will refrain from translating the word *kami* into English. In one sense the term refers to the deities or gods that are associated with the Shintō pantheon, but it can also refer to the ephemeral quality of the world or nature in a more abstract sense than reference to specific deities or the pantheon. See Nelson (1996:256) for a clear definition of the concept.

3. Love, of course, is not a concept that is neutral with respect to culture. The meaning of love varies. The manner in which love is conceptualized in the Japanese context is an area for which there is considerable room for further research. For an ethnographic discussion of love see Hamabata 1990 and for an emic perspective see Asahi Shinbunsha 1997.

4. The expression of concern for the dead in relation to the nation is readily evident in the visits of Prime Ministers to Yasukuni Shrine to commemorate the war dead who are enshrined there as "ancestral *kami*" (http://www.yasukuni.or.jp/english/). The web site for Yasukuni shrine offers the nationalistic explanation of those enshrined there in the statement that: "The noble souls who are worshiped at Yasukuni offered up their lives with deep love for their families, their race and their nation. With heartfelt thoughts for the increasing prosperity of generations and generations to come of their families, relatives and their fellow countrymen, these noble souls endured hardships and offered even their lives for the sake of their nation and race" (http://www.yasukuni.or.jp/english/). For a good discussion of Yasukuni, see Hardacre 1989.

5. There are some forms of religious belonging in Japan that do involve exclusivity, such as Jehovah's Witness and the Buddhism-

based new religion Sōka Gakkai (among other new religions). For a very useful discussion of one new religion see Hardacre (1984). Faith does also play a role in some more traditional religions such as Shin Buddhism, which has been compared to Lutheranism in the emphasis on faith alone as a means to salvation (Andreasen 1998:11). However, the fact that the institutional religion emphasizes faith and salvation does not necessarily mean that participants place a great deal of emphasis on these concerns.

6. For an excellent study of the manner in which a Japanese conjugal pair conceptualize sacred space and entities, see Roberts, Morita, and Brown (1986).

7. The name Yamada is a pseudonym for the actual hamlet.

8. It is important to note that this form of family organization exists in varying degrees in different parts of Japan. In rural areas such as Tōhoku, for example, it is not uncommon to find this structure, or to encounter people who are aware of this structure as having occurred in the history of one's family, even if this is not considered an important aspect of the current family organization.

9. For example, upon leaving one's home, a person will normally say "*ite kimasu*," although one can also use the more formal "*ite mairimasu.*"

10. It is interesting to note that the amount of time that food stays on the *butsudan* can vary considerably. Perishable food may be placed briefly on the *butsudan* and then removed to a refrigerator, while packaged foods may be left on the *butsudan* for a few days.

11. These data were collected by Blaine Connor, who worked as my research assistant during the summer of 2000.

Chapter 5

1. Tanka poem written by Itoh Setsuko. *Naki hito mo genshin no hito mo kubetsu naku yume ni dete kuru aki no yo nagashi.* Translation mine.

2. These data were collected in an interview conducted by Blaine Connor as part of the project on religion, well-being, and aging in Japan funded by the National Institute on Aging, John Traphagan, Principal Investigator, AG016111.

3. One man in his seventies stated, "my wife passed away, but I still can see her in my dreams, and my mother has had similar dreams." When asked about the meaning of these dreams, this man responded that it might be simply because he wants to see her again, or "because my body is tired and old." Like many other men, this informant was hesitant to place the experience of dreams into the framework of ancestral protection.

4. Although, in this chapter I will discuss the experiences of dreams among a small group of women from Akita Prefecture, I have encountered similar dream experiences in Iwate Prefecture and there is a general perception that the appearance of ancestors in dreams is common. Indeed, when told that some people in Yamada had seen their ancestors in their dreams, two women nodded and said, "Yes, yes. Not just in Yamada, [this happens all over Japan]."

5. As I have noted elsewhere (Traphagan 2003b:132), the importance of dreams of ancestors is nothing new in Japan. Throughout Japanese literature, one can find numerous references to the appearance of the dead in dreams and the importance of interpreting those experiences in terms of their meaning in the world of the living. In the 11th Century novel *The Tale of Genji*, for instance, the young emperor who has banished Genji to another part of Japan experiences feelings of guilt because the banishment contradicts the wishes of his deceased father, as revealed in a dream in which his father visits him, an experience that leads him to summon Genji to return (Puette 1983:90). Other characters in the novel, including Genji are visited by ancestors in dreams; Genji is visited by his dead father who offers him advice, and by a deceased lover who chastises him for his behavior with a woman (Puette 1983:97). Dreams are often interpreted by the characters in *Genji* as being forms of commentary on the behavior of the living, or as advice from the dead on how to decide on courses of action. In recent forms of literature and film, the dead sometimes appear to consult with or advise the living. For example, Kurosawa's film *Dreams*, contains one vignette in which the spirits of deceased soldiers appear to their commander, who alone among his platoon has survived World War II. When the first dead soldier, Noguchi, appears, the commander informs him that, in fact, he did really die along with the rest of his

platoon. As the entire platoon marches before him, he implores them to return to their world rather than haunting the world of the living. Noguchi looks off into the distant valley lamenting the fact that his parents await his return, unaware that he is truly dead. There is a sense in this scene of the sadness about the disconnection between the living and the dead and at least a tacit feeling that the communication between the dead and the living is one in which not only do the dead watch over the living, but the living may, in fact, be able to help the dead find rest. See Rimer (1976) for an interesting example in which women and dreams are associated in a play by Tanaka Chikao.

6. It is important to recognize that the experience of ancestral visitation in dreams is by no means unique to Japanese culture (see also Traphagan 2003b:132). Malinowski, for example, noted during World War I that in the Trobriand Islands spirits (*baloma*) of dead relatives sometimes appeared to the living in dreams immediately after death and visited the living in dreams during the annual feast (Malinowski 1916:66). In more recent work Lutz reports that among the Ifaluk in Micronesia spirits sometimes visit the living in dreams and people are chased, frightened, or disaster occurs in the life of a family member, with people discussing the meanings of such dreams the following morning. Specific spirits are associated with illness and discussions arise as to determining which spirit has caused a threat and how to go about curing that threat (Lutz 1988:93). While many of these dreams are bad omens, Lutz notes that not all dreams in which spirits appear are negatively interpreted, but also may be interpreted as an indication of good fortune to come for the household (Lutz 1988:242). Dreams have also been reported as evidence of spirit possession in Northern Sudan (Boddy 1989), and variations in the content of dreams have been noted between men and women (Colby 1963). Strathern discusses dream interpretation among the Melpa of Papua New Guinea as being derived from a set of symbols and associated meanings that form a "code for translating the obscurities of dreams" into what they signify, even while the particular interpretations of dreams vary and often depend upon and correspond to the perspectives of those involved (Strathern 1989:314). Furthermore, Lohmann (2000) has explored the manner in which dream encoun-

ters with supernatural beings among the Asabano of Papua New Guinea provide evidence of both their existence and power an observation that, as will be shown below, has relevance for the study of ancestral dreams in Japan. See Eggan (1952, 1961) and Kuper (1979) for discussions of dreams and dream analysis in anthropology.

7. It is certainly possible that this role as caretaker of familial well-being is closely tied to the gendered expression of power within the family, in which the domain of female-centered power is structured around the use of expressing concern as a way to manage kin relationships and exercise influence over other family members (cf. Strathern 1989:304). While I have encountered instances, one of which is included here, in which older women have reported dreams to family members as a way of alerting them to potential danger, I do not have specific data that indicate women use these dream experiences to manipulate family members' behavior.

8. These dream cases are also discussed in Traphagan (2003b). Interviews in which dreams were discussed were conducted with approximately 50 men and women over the age of 65.

9. *Watashi ga so yappa shi sō iu nakunatta hito ga ano yume no naka ni deta toki wa, ano yappari kazoku to ka shimpai shite kureta ka na to omimasu.*

10. As noted above, in this study, although men did sometimes report the appearance of ancestors in dreams, in general it was women who had such experiences and who were more inclined to interpret these experiences in terms of protection. One man, for instance, stated that he had experienced his mother (*jibun no hahaoya*) coming into a dream (*yume ni hairimashita*). In this case it was difficult to determine the man's interpretation of the dream. He stated at one point that the particular meaning was that he wanted to see his mother (*mitai to wake mitai...*). Interestingly, he went on to indicate that, like the man discussed in note 3, his body was tired due to his age (80) and, although not making a direct connection, ended the conversation with "*mukae ni kuru ka*" indicating that he is close to death (literally to be taken away).

11. This should not be taken as suggesting that Japanese privilege this approach over biomedical approaches to understanding disease.

Rather, both are used in a complimentary way. Most Japanese will visit a doctor and accept a biomedical definition of and solution to their ailment, but issues of harmony and balance also are important to how people think about the health of mind and body.

12. The case of the Black Carib women about whom Virginia Kerns writes is quite similar to my findings among older Japanese women. For Black Carib women on the island of St. Vincent in the West Indies, both on ritual occasions and within the more mundane context of daily life, "older women act together to sustain moral and social order" through which they carry out "their lifelong responsibility to protect and care for their children and other lineal kin" (Kerns 1997:5). Early in life, as daughters and mothers, women care for their children and for aging parents, and following the death of their parents, they are the ones responsible for organizing the appropriate rituals (Kerns 1997:107). The central role of a woman within Black Carib culture is that of caregiver — whether it is to one's children or to elder parents. Older women, according to Kerns, often attribute good health in their children to having faithfully attended to the dead through appropriate rituals — to neglect the ancestors is to invite illness or other misfortune upon a woman's children. And carrying out appropriate rituals is one way of caring for one's children through caring for one's ancestors. As in the cases from Japan I have discussed here, for at least one of the women that Kerns interviews dreams were a context in which communication with the ancestors occurred, specifically in the form of requests for offerings (Kerns 1997:177).

13. The questionnaire was administered to 95 percent of the people over the age of 60 who were living in the hamlet of Jōnai in 1996. My aim was to obtain a 100 percent sample in the sampling universe (the hamlet), although some potential participants were either unable (due to health) or unwilling to participate. The questionnaire included questions on a broad range of issues related to the elderly, including subjective reporting of health status, income levels, and attitudes about aging and how the elderly are perceived. It might be argued that since the questionnaire was directed at the elderly it is skewed because they are inclined to respond that they, themselves, are the most involved in doing ancestral rituals. While this may be

the case, extensive observation of who does ancestral rituals in several families in both Iwate and Akita support the results of the questionnaire.

14. Of course, if one looks at the role of women historically, it is clear that they have typically had a generalized caregiver role in that they are expected to manage most aspects of the household and care for whomever needs care within the household (see Bernstein 1983). To some extent the shift to a more compartmentalized approach to caregiving may be related to tendencies in modern society in which women are typically expected to stay home and care for children while husbands work. In farm and merchant families in Kanegasaki, women may work while also being responsible for raising the children. In one merchant family, the husband and wife manage two beauty salons. The husband manages one located in a neighboring city while the wife remains at the one in Kanegasaki, which is in the same building where the family lives. This allows her to work while also being in close proximity to her children on a daily basis. In many three-generation families in Kanegasaki, the woman in the middle generation (the *yome*) may work while Grandma (or sometimes Grandpa) takes care of the children. This pattern typically changes abruptly when a member of the elder generation becomes ill. In most cases, a woman will quit her job in order to provide care for a member of the elder generation when the need arises.

15. It is worth noting that when confronted with this hypothesis, one informant, a man in his sixties, disagreed with my conclusion. His take on this was that, "at the moment, I think it is because women live longer, so they are more likely to become demented. The dreams come out in relation to their demented state and because there are more elderly women than men, it seems as though there are more of them having dreams of this sort. But it is a product of Alzheimer's disease or other forms of dementia. Maybe it is a result of brain atrophy."

16. It is interesting to note that the categories of "healing" roles available to older women in Japan have similarities with those described by Sargent in Benin (Sargent 1991:211).

Chapter 6

1. As I have argued elsewhere (Traphagan 2000c), the Kanegasaki festival forms a framework through which people enact social relations—particularly those related to age hierarchies—and represent these social relations in a visible, public way (Douglas 1966:128, see also Schnell 1999:234). Partly due to its administrative location within an age grade system structured around the gerontocratic political organization of area neighborhoods, the festival serves the function of representing and reproducing the age hierarchy—which, at least from a rhetorical perspective, places the elderly in a position of high status in the community—that exists in local neighborhoods. However, as Hazan (1994:54) notes, it is common in urbanized societies for the status of the elderly to be equivocal, and this is no different in Japan. Much as the festival itself is met with a degree of ambivalence by younger members of the community, the status of the elderly, too, is equivocally defined—at once being represented as powerful and important and at the same time obsolete and even resented.

2. The *mikoshi* for which I was one of the carriers during the 1996 *kabōsai* festival consists of four long pieces of wood set in a tic-tac-toe cross fashion to serve as handles. The *mikoshi* houses the deity of the shrine and, thus, is the vehicle through which its supernatural presence is placed directly into contact with the community (Schnell 1995:308). On top of the central square is a platform on which is mounted a *komodaru*, a 72 liter barrel for saké that is empty of saké, although it has been weighted down to make the task of carrying it more arduous (see Figure 6.2). On top of the barrel is affixed the object that informants involved in the festival referred to as the *kami-sama* (a formal term for a Shintō deity), which is a piece of wood to which is attached a white piece of paper from the main Shinto shrine in Kanegasaki. Along the inside square are placed drapes of red cloth to cover the boards used for holding the saké barrel up and the handle areas are wrapped with cloth so that they form an alternating red and white pattern. These colors are common in Japanese celebrations. In front of the *mikoshi* two children—in 1996 two identical twin girls

who were 5 years old—walk carrying baskets full of salt. They spread
the salt on the road to purify the area directly in front of *mikoshi* before it passes.

3. I have discussed the manner in which this system has similarities to both age grades and age sets in Traphagan 1998c and 2000a.

4. Old Persons Club is a direct translation of *rōjin kurabu.*

5. It is important to note that these age grade associations are local
organizations and are differentiated from the national system of
seinenkai and *fujinkai* that also exist in parallel to these local groups. One
can also find *seinenkai* and *fujinkai* associated with agricultural cooper-
atives in farming areas, as well as business organizations in merchant
districts. It is not unusual for a person to belong to more than one similar association at the same time, particularly when it involves one's
neighborhood association and an association related to one's work.

6. Data on the Kanto Matsuri were collected by Hitoko Nakamura,
who worked as my research assistant during the summer of 2000.

7. *Pachinko* is a form of gambling that is extremely popular in
Japan. It involves machines that are similar to pinball machines and
is played in large buildings with banks of such machines.

8. It might be argued that the ritual only manifestly reinforces the
social position of elder males as powerful, while presenting a public
illusion of that power as other, younger members of society wield
power. This is far from the case in agricultural Japan where, as noted
earlier, virtually all positions of political power within neighborhoods
are held by elder men. This is not to argue that younger men have no
power. In governmental institutions such as the Town Hall, they do.
But within the immediate context of neighborhood leadership and
control, it is the elder men who make decisions and guide younger
men in the execution of rituals and other neighborhood activities. Indeed, most meetings held to discuss issues of neighborhood politics
are held during the day, when younger men are away at work. Of
course, these men do have influence within the contexts of their
households when talking to elder family members, but the decision-
making is almost entirely within the hands of elder men.

9. In *kabōsai,* the focus of the ritual performance of concern rests
upon those who are twenty-five. Only these individuals are able to

participate specifically as *yakudoshi*, although there may be other members of performance groups in the festival who happen to be in *yakudoshi* during a given year. The specific way in which the *yakudoshi* group chooses to participate is up to them. Usually it involves wearing home-made costumes (anything from clown suits to the more traditional *happi* coats commonly worn at festivals in Japan) and dancing as the procession moves through the town. I have never been able to obtain an explanation as to why the participation of *yakudoshi* in this festival is limited to those at age twenty-five.

Chapter 7

1. *Shukubō no yume ni dete kuru tomo odoru, samereba ame ga noku no ishi utsu.*

2. It is important to note that in the anthropological literature, religion and magic have long been viewed as separate. Unlike religious rituals, those associated with magic do not involve spiritual agencies, but instead are concerned with the manipulation by humans of various "powers" to achieve specific results. Durkheim (1965) notes these differences, and Frazer emphasizes the practical aspects of magic in contrast to religious rituals (1998). For a useful introduction to this see Hicks (1999:257–258).

3. Again, this is not limited to Japan. In Korea, male-centered rituals associated with both Confucianism and ancestor veneration may be practiced in the same household, along with female-centered shamanistic rituals (Kendall 1985).

4. See Good (1994:14–24) for a very clear discussion of the importance of the work of Evans-Pritchard for medical anthropology. Good's discussion of Evans-Pritchard's approach to the issue of belief has influenced my thinking on the subject here.

Glossary of Key Terms

Terms that can begin with the honorific "o" are categorized under "o," as these are normally used in this way.

amae	Dependence
amaeru	To depend, with *amae* implies a sense of interdependence
amayakasu	To indulge another's dependence; with *amaeru* implies a sense of interdependence
arutsuhaimā	Alzheimer's disease
bekke	Branch family without kinship ties
boke	Indigenous Japanese concept related to senility or senile dementia (see Traphagan 2000a)
boke rōjin	Senile old person
bunke	Branch family with kinship ties
butsudan	Buddhist family altar
byōki	Sickness, illness
danka	Temple parish
ema	Votive tables on which people write messages and requests to the deities
fujinbu	Women's Association
fujinkai	Women's Association
furui	Old, obsolete

go	Japanese board game
(go)senzo	Ancestor(s)
hamaya	Arrow used for driving away evil spirits
honke	Stem or main family
hotoke	Ancestors, Buddha
ie	House, household, family
ihai	Mortuary tablet
ikigai	One's purpose in life, *raison d'être*
inaka	Relative term used to indicate rural as opposed to urban areas
jichikai	Self-Government Association
jinja	Shintō shrine
jōdo shinshū	Pure Land sect of Buddhism
kabōsai	Fire prevention festival
kachikan	Values
kaimyō	Posthumous name given by Buddhist priest at the time of the funeral
kami(-sama)	Deities associated with Shintō
kamidana	Shintō family altar, god shelf
kampō	East Asian medicine
kanjō	Emotions
kanreki	60th birthday, marked by giving a red sweater; marks the transition from middle age to old age and rebirth into a new phase of life
kazoku	Family, typically the nuclear family
kenkō	Health
kodomokai	Children's Association
kokoro	Heart, mind, center
kōminkan	Community center

komodaru	Cask of sake wrapped in straw
koseki	Family register
magobunke	A branch of a branch family
mamoru	To protect
matsuri	Festival, often associated with a Shintō shrine
mikan	Mandarin oranges
miko	Shrine maiden
mikoshi	Palanquin or portable shrine
mizuko kuyō	Ritual for aborted fetuses, miscarriages, and still borns
muenbotoke	Unattached spirits of the dead
mukoyōshi	Adoptive male brought in as successor to a family either without a son or without a competent or willing son to take on the headship of the household
myōjin	Shrine/deity often placed at the northwest corner of one's property
netakiri rōjin	Bed-ridden old person
nembutsu	Recitation of the name of Amida
nisetai jūtaku	Housing arrangement in which multiple generations of the same family occupy a single building while keeping separate living areas
obon	Summer festival of the dead
ogamu	To pray
ohaka	Grave, collective family grave
ohigan	Vernal or autumnal equinox
omairi	Prayer, visiting a temple, gravesite, or shrine
omamori	Talismans
omiyamairi	Ritual for newborns
omochi	Pounded rice cakes

omukae	Literally to be met and greeted, often used as a way of referring to death by the elderly to indicate being taken away by the ancestors
onegai (suru)	To request something
onna rashii	Feminine (stereotypically)
oshimotsuki	Period commemorating the death of Shinran
oya kōkō	Filial piety, refers to the showing of concern and caring for parents and appropriate behavior vis-à-vis parents
pokkuri-dera	A Buddhist temple at which people pray for a sudden or quick death, devoid of prolonged illness and the associated pain and embarassment of becoming a burden by requiring care
rengōkai	Unity Association, in Kanegasaki it includes the heads of the Self-Government Associations for a district
rōjin	Old person, the elderly
rōjin kurabu	Old Persons Club(s)
rōjinsei chihō	Senile dementia (from a biomedical perspective)
sakaki	Branches from the sakaki tree (cleyera japonica) considered a sacred tree in Shintō
sake	Rice wine
seijinshiki	Coming-of-age ceremony at 20 that involves a visit to a shrine
seinenbu	Young Men's Association
seinenkai	Young Person Association, sometimes limited to men
sekihan	Rice with red beans, eaten at auspicious occasions
sensei	Literally teacher, but can refer to any person of high status, such as doctors, lawyers, or politicians
shichi-go-san	Ceremony at shrine for girls at age 3 and 7 and boys at age 5

shikata ga nai	There's nothing one can do
soto	Outside
suijin	Shrine/deity to protect the well at a house
susuharai	Year-end cleaning of one's house on New Year's Eve
taiyaku	Ages of major calamity, normally 33 for women and 42 for men
tatami	Straw mats used to cover the floor in many Japanese houses
tera	Buddhist temple
tokonoma	Alcove in which art objects are often placed
torii	Gate typically found at the entrance or along a path leading to a Shintō shrine
yakudoshi	Inauspicious years in the lifecourse
yatai	Float used in festivals
yome	Bride, young wife, a woman brought into her husband's natal household where she will co-reside (although this is not necessarily the case)

Bibliography

Adelson, Naomi. 2000. *'Being Alive Well': Health and the Politics of Cree Well-Being*. Toronto: University of Toronto Press.

Allison, Anne. 1994. *Nightwork: Sexuality, Pleasure, and Corporate Masculinity in a Tokyo Hostess Club*. University of Chicago Press.

Alter, Joe. 1999. Heaps of Health, Metaphysical Fitness: Ayurveda and the Ontology of Good Health in Medical Anthropology. *Current Anthropology* 40(S1):S43–S66.

Anandarajah, G. and Hight E. 2001. Spirituality and Medical Practice: Using the HOPE Questions as a Practical Tool for Spiritual Assessment. *American Family Physician* 63(1):81–89.

Andreason, Esben. 1998. *Popular Buddhism in Japan: Shin Buddhist Religion and Culture*. Honolulu: University of Hawaii Press.

Ariyoshi Sawako. 1972. *Kōkotsu no hito*. Tokyo: Shinchosha.

Ariyoshi Sawako. 1987. *The Twilight Years*. Mildred Tahara, trans. New York: Kodansha International.

Aruga, Kizaemon. 1954. The Family in Japan. *Marriage and Family Living* 16:362–368.

Asahi Shinbun Atkia Shikyoku [Asahi Newspaper Akita Branch Office], ed. 2000. *Jisatsu: jisatsuritsu zenkoku—Akita kara no hōkoku* [Suicide: National Suicide Rates—Report from Akita]. Akita: Mumyōsha shuppan.

Asahi Shinbun Online. 2003. Diet OKs Legislation Urging Repopulation. http://www.asahi.com/english/politics/K2003072400272.html. July 24th.

Asahi Shinbunsha. 1997. *Ren'ai to Kekkon: Meiji, Taishō*. Tokyo: Asahi Shinbunsha.

Ashkenazi, Michael. 1993. *Matsuri: Festival of a Japanese Town*. Honolulu: University of Hawaii Press.

Baer, Hans A. 2001. *Biomedicine and Alternative Healing Systems in America: Issues of Class, Race, Ethnicity, and Gender*. Madison: University of Wisconsin Press.

Beardsley, Richard K., John W. Hall, and Robert E. Ward. 1959. *Village Japan*. Chicago: The University of Chicago Press.

Befu, Harumi. 1963. Patrilineal Descent and Personal Kindred in Japan. *American Anthropologist* 95(6):1328–1341

Befu, Harumi. 1968. Gift-Giving in a Modernizing Japan. *Monumenta Nipponica* 23(3/4):445–456.

Befu, Harumi. 1993. An Ethnography of Dinner Entertainment in Japan. In Subhash Durlabhji and Norton E. Marks (eds.), *Japanese Business: Cultural Perspectives* (pp. 123–140). Albany: State University of New York Press.

Bell, Catherine. 1992. *Ritual Theory, Ritual Practice*. New York: Oxford University Press.

Bergson, Henri. 1990 [1962]. *Matter and Memory*. N., M. Paul and W. S. Palmer, trans. London: Zone Books.

Bernstein, Gail Lee. 1983. *Haruko's World: A Japanese Farm Woman and Her Community*. Stanford: Stanford University Press.

Bestor, Theodore C. 1989. *Neighborhood Tokyo*. Stanford: Stanford University Press.

Bix, Herbert P. 2000. *Hirohito and the Making of Modern Japan*. New York: HarperCollins.

Blacker, Carmen. 1975. *The Catalpa Bow: A Study of Shamanistic Practices in Japan*. London: George Allen and Unwin.

Bloch, Maurice. 1989. *Ritual, History, and Power*. London: The Athlone Press.

Bloom, Alfred. 1965. *Shinran's Gospel of Pure Grace*. Tuscon: The University of Arizona Press.

Boddy, Janice. 1989. *Wombs and Alien Spirits: Women, Men, and the Zār Cult in Northern Sudan.* Madison: University of Wisconsin Press.

Bourdieu, Pierre. 1977. *Outline of a Theory of Practice.* Richard Nice, trans. New York: Cambridge University Press.

Bourdieu, Pierre. 1990. *The Logic of Practice.* Richard Nice, trans. Stanford: Stanford University Press.

Brown, Keith. 1966. Dōzoku and Descent Ideology in Japan. *American Anthropologist* 68:1129–1151.

Brown, Keith. 1968. The Content of Dōzoku Relationships in Japan. *Ethnology* 7(2):113–138.

Brown, Keith, trans. 1979. *Shinjō: The Chronicle of a Japanese Village.* Pittsburgh: University Center for International Studies, University of Pittsburgh.

Brown, Keith. 1980. The Family in Japan. World Conference on Records, August 12–15.

Brown, Naomi. 2003. Under One Roof: The Evolving Story of Three Generation Housing in Japan. In John W. Traphagan and John Knight (eds.) *Demographic Change and the Family in Japan's Aging Society.* Albany: The State University of New York Press.

Bumiller, Elisabeth. 1995. *The Secrets of Mariko: A Year in the Life of a Japanese Woman and Her Family.* New York: Vintage Books.

Bunkachō (Ministry of Cultural Affairs), (ed.) 1995. *Shūkyō Nenkan* (Religion Yearbook). Tokyo: Gyōsei.

Cetina, Karen Knorr. 1999. *Epistemic Cultures: How the Sciences Make Knowledge.* Cambridge: Harvard University Press.

Clark, Scott. 1994. *Japan: A View from the Bath.* Honolulu: University of Hawaii Press.

Cohen, Lawrence. 1998. *No Aging in India: Alzheimer's, the Bad Family, and Other Modern Things.* Berkeley: University of California Press.

Colby, Kenneth M. 1963. Sex Differences in Dreams of Primitive Tribes. *American Anthropologist* 65:1116–1112.

Connerton, Paul. 1989. *How Societies Remember*. New York: Cambridge University Press.

Constable, Nicole. 1997. *Maid to Order in Hong Kong: Stories of Filipina Workers*. Ithaca: Cornell University Press.

Creighton, Millie. 1997. Consuming Rural Japan: The Marketing of Tradition and Nostalgia in the Japanese Travel Industry. *Ethnology* 36(3):239–254.

Davis, Winston B. 1980. *Dojo: Magic and Exorcism in Modern Japan*. Stanford: Stanford University Press.

Davis, Winston B. 1992. *Japanese Religion and Society: Paradigms of Structure and Change*. Albany: State University of New York Press.

Doi, Takeo. 1973. *The Anatomy of Dependence*. New York: Kodansha.

Douglas, Mary. 1966. *Purity and Danger: An Analysis of Concepts of Pollution and Taboo*. London: Routledge and Kegan Paul.

Durkheim, Emile. 1965 [1915]. *The Elementary Forms of the Religious Life*. New York: The Free Press.

Earhart, H. Byron. 1989. *Gedatsu-kai and Religion in Contemporary Japan: Returning to the Center*. Bloomington: Indiana University Press.

Eggan, Dorothy. 1952. The Manifest Content of Dreams: A Challenge to Social Science. *American Anthropologist* 54(4):469–485.

Eggan, Dorothy. 1961. Dream Analysis. In *Studying Personality Cross-Culturally*. Bert Kaplan, ed. Evanston: Row, Peterson.

Embree, John T. 1964 [1939]. *Suye Mura: A Japanese Village*. Chicago: University of Chicago Press.

Evans-Pritchard, E. E. 1940. *The Nuer*. New York: Oxford University Press.

Evans-Pritchard, 1976[1937]. *Witchcraft, Oracles, and Magic among the Azande*. Oxford: Clarendon Press.

Flood, Gavin. 1996. *An Introduction to Hinduism*. New York: Cambridge University Press.

Fortes, Meyer. 1984. Age, Generation, and Social Structure. In *Age and Anthropological Theory*, edited by David I. Kertzer and Jennie Keith. Pp. 99–122. Ithaca: Cornell University Press.

Foucault, Michel. 1977. *Discipline and Punish: Birth of a Prison*. Alan Sheridan, trans. New York: Pantheon Books.

Foucault, Michel. 1978. *The History of Sexuality: An Introduction, Vol. 1*. Robert Hurley, trans. New York: Vintage Books.

Frazer, James George. 1998. *The Golden Bough: A Study in Magic and Religion*. Oxford: Oxford University Press (abridgement of 2nd and 3rd editions).

Fujishima, Gaijirō. 1961. *Hiraizumi: Mōtsuji to Kanjizaiōin no Kenkyū* [*Hiraizumi: A Study on Mōtsu-ji Temple and Kanjizaiō-in Temple*]. Tōkyō: Tōkyō Daigaku Shuppankai.

Fukurai, Hiroshi. 1991. Japanese Migration in Contemporary Japan: Economic Segmentation and Interprefectural Migration. *Social Biology* 38(1–2):28–50.

Geertz, Clifford. 1973. *The Interpretation of Cultures*. New York: Basic Books.

Geertz, Clifford. 1983. *Local Knowledge*. New York: Basic Books.

Gill, Tom. 2001. *Men of Uncertainty: The Social Organization of Day Laborers in Contemporary Japan*. Albany: The State University of New York Press.

Gonda, Takashi. No date. *Kashikoi obā-chan no boke yobō doku hon* [Wise Grandma's *Boke* Prevention Reader]. Tokyo: Nihon kādo kōgeisha.

Good, Byron J. 1994. *Medicine, Rationality, and Experience: An Anthropological Perspective*. New York: Cambridge University Press.

Gramsci. 1971. Selections from Cultural Writings. William Boelhower, trans. Cambridge: Harvard University Press.

Grimes, Ronald L. 1982. *Beginnings in Ritual Studies*. New York: University Press of America.

Guthrie, Stewart. 1988. *A Japanese New Religion: Risshō Kōsei-kai in a Mountain Hamlet*. Ann Arbor: University of Michigan Center for Japanese Studies.

Haley, Katherine C., Harold G. Koenig, and Bruce M. Burchett. 2001. Relationship Between Private Religious Activity and Physical Functioning in Older Adults. *Journal of Religion and Health* 40(2):305–312.

Hamabata, Matthews Masayuki. 1990. *Crested Kimono: Power and Love in the Japanese Business Family*. Ithaca: Cornell University Press.

Hardacre, Helen. 1984. Lay Buddhism in Contemporary Japan: Reiyukai Kyodan. Princeton: Princeton University Press.

Hardacre, Helen. 1989. *Shintō and the State 1868–1988*. Princeton: Princeton University Press.

Hardacre, Helen. 1997. *Marketing the Menacing Fetus in Japan*. Berkeley: University of California Press.

Harris, Phyllis Braudy, Susan Orpett Long, and Miwa Fujii. 1998. Men and Elder Care in Japan: A Ripple of Change? *Journal of Cross-Cultural Gerontology* 13(2):177–198.

Hashimoto, Akiko. 1996. *The Gift of Generations: Japanese and American Perspectives on Aging and the Social Contract*. New York: Cambridge University Press.

Haviland, William A. 1999. *Cultural Anthropology, 9th Edition*. New York: Harcourt Brace College Publishers.

Hazan, Haim. 1994. *Old Age Constructions and Deconstructions*. New York: Cambridge University Press.

Hendry, Joy. 1981. Tomodachi Kō: Age-Mate Groups in Northern Kyushu. *Proceedings of the British Association of Japanese Studies* 6:44–56.

Hicks, David, ed. 1999. *Ritual and Belief: Readings in the Anthropology of Religion*. New York: McGraw-Hill.

Hornum, Barbara. 1995. Assessing Types of Residential Accomodations for the Elderly: Liminality and Communitas. In J. Neil

Henderson and Maria Vesperi (eds.), *The Culture of Long-Term Care*. Westport, CT: Bergin and Garvey.

Imamura, Anne E. 1987. *Urban Japanese Housewives: At Home and in the Community*. Honolulu: University of Hawaii Press.

John E. Fetzer Institute. 1999. *Multidimensional Measurement of Religiousness/Spirituality for Use in Health Research*. Kalamazoo, MI: John E. Fetzer Institute.

Johnson, Mark. 1987. *The Body in the Mind: The Bodily Basis of Meaning, Imagination, and Reason*. Chicago: University of Chicago Press.

Kawano, Satsuki. 1996. Gender, Liminality and Ritual in Japan: Divination among Single Tokyo Women. *Journal of Ritual Studies* 9:65–91.

Kendall, Laurel. 1985. *Shamans, Housewives, and Other Restless Spirits*. Honolulu: University of Hawaii Press.

Kerns, Virginia. 1997. *Women and the Ancestors: Black Carib Kinship and Ritual, 2nd Edition*. Urbana: University of Illinois Press.

Ketelaar, James Edward. 1990. *Of Heretics and Martyrs in Meiji Japan: Buddhism and Its Persecution*. Princeton: Princeton University Press.

Kiefer, Christie W. 1999. "Autonomy and Stigma in Aging Japan," In *Lives in Motion: Composing Circles of Self and Community in Japan*, edited by Susan Orpett Long. Ithaca: Cornell East Asia Series.

Kikkawa, Takehiko. 1995. *Hito wa naze bokeru no ka: boke no genin to keā* [Why Do People Become *Boke*? The Causes and Care of *Boke*]. Tokyo: Shinseidehansha.

Kinoshita, Yasuhito and Christie W. Kiefer. 1992. *Refuge of the Honored: Social Organization in a Japanese Retirement Community*. Berkeley: University of California Press.

Kitagawa, Joseph M. 1966. *Religion in Japanese History*. New York: Columbia University Press.

Koenig, Harold G. 1995. Religion and Health in Later Life. In *Aging, Spirituality, and Religion: A Handbook*, edited by Melvin A. Kimble, et al. Minneapolis: Fortress Press.

Kondo, Dorinne K. 1990. *Crafting Selves: Power, Gender, and Discourses of Identity in a Japanese Workplace*. Chicago: University of Chicago Press.

Krause, Neal and Berit Ingersoll-Dayton. 1999. Religion, Social Support, and Health among Japanese Elderly. *Journal of Health and Social Behavior* 40(4):405–424.

Krause, Neal. et al. 2002. Religion, Death of a Loved One, and Hypertension among Older Adults in Japan. *Journal of Gerontology B: Psychological and Social Sciences* 57(2):S96–S107.

Kuper, Adam. 1979. A Structural Approach to Dreams. *Man* (N.S.) 14:645–662.

Kurosu, Satomi. 1991. Suicide in Rural Areas: The Case of Japan 1960–1980. *Rural Sociology* 56(4):603–618.

LaFleur, William R. 1992. *Liquid Life: Abortion and Buddhism in Japan*. Princeton: Princeton University Press.

Lebra, Takie Sugiyama. 1976. *Japanese Patterns of Behavior*. Honolulu: University of Hawaii Press.

Lebra, Takie Sugiyama. 1986. *Japanese Women: Constraint and Fulfillment*. Honolulu: University of Hawaii Press.

Lebra, Takie Sugiyama. 1993. *Above the Clouds: Status Culture of the Modern Japanese Nobility*. Berkeley: University of California Press.

Lévi-Strauss, Claude. 1974. *Structural Anthropology*. Claire Jacobson and Broke Grundfest Schoepf, trans. New York: Basic Books.

Liaw, Kao-Lee. 1992. Interprefectural Migration and its Effects on Prefectural Populations in Japan: An Analysis Based on the 1980 Census. *The Canadian Geographer* 36(4):320–35.

Lipp, Frank J. 1991. *The Mixe of Oaxaca: Religion, Ritual, and Healing*. Austin: University of Texas Press.

Lock, Margaret M. 1980. *East Asian Medicine in Urban Japan: Varieties of Medical Experience*. Berkeley: University of California Press.

Lock, Margaret. 1993. *Encounters with Aging: Mythologies of Menopause in Japan and North America*. Berkeley: University of California Press.

Lohmann, Rover Ivar. 2000. The Role of Dreams in Religious Enculturation among the Asabano of Papua New Guinea. *Ethos* 28(1):75–102.

Long, Susan O. 1997. Reflections on Becoming a Cucumber: Images of the Good Death in Japan and the U.S. Unpublished Paper Presented at the Center for Japanese Studies, University of Michigan.

Long, Susan O. 1999. *Shikata Ga Nai*: Resignation, Control, and Self-Identity. In *Lives in Motion: Composing circles of self and community in Japan*. Edited by Susan O. Long. Ithaca: Cornell East Asia Series.

Long, Susan O. 2003. Becoming a Cucumber: Culture, Nature, and the Good Death in Japan and the United States. *Journal of Japanese Studies* 29(1):33–69.

Lutz, Catherine A. 1988. *Unnatural Emotions: Everyday Sentiments on a Micronesian Atoll and Their Challenge to Western Theory*. Chicago: University of Chicago Press.

Lyotard, Jean-François. 1984. *The Postmodern Condition: A Report on Knowledge*. Geoff Bennington and Brian Masumi, transl. Minneapolis: University of Minnesota Press.

Malinowski, Bronislaw. 1916. Baloma; The Spirits of the Dead in the Trobriand Islands. *Journal of the Royal Anthropological Institute of Great Britain and Ireland* 46:353–430.

Margenau, Henry. 1977[1950]. *The Nature of Physical Reality*. Woodbridge, CT: Ox Bow Press.

Markides, K.S., J.S. Levin & L.A. Ray. 1987. Religion, Aging, and Life Satisfaction: An Eight-Year, Three-Wave Longitudinal Study. *The Gerontologist* 25:660–665.

Mathews, Gordon. 1996. *What Makes Life Worth Living? How Japanese and Americans Make Sense of Their Worlds.* Berkeley: University of California Press.

Matsumoto, Toshiaki. 1995. *Rōnenki no jisatsu ni kansuru jisshōteki kenkyū* [Research Providing Conclusive Evidence for Suicide in Old Age]. Tokyo: Taga shuppan kabushiki kaisha.

McFadden, S.H. 1995. Religion and Well-Being in Aging Persons in an Aging Society. *Journal of Social Issues* 51, 161–175.

Miller, James. 1965. Living Systems: Basic Concepts. *Behavioral Science* 10(3):193–257.

Mullins, Mark. 1998. *Christianity Made in Japan: A Study of Indigenous Movements.* Honolulu: University of Hawaii Press.

Musick, Marc, John W. Traphagan, Harold Koenig, David Larson. 2000. Spirituality and Physical Health in Aging. *Journal of Adult Development* 7(2):73–86.

Nakane, Chie. 1967. *Kinship and Economic Organization in Rural Japan.* New York: Academic Press.

Nakata, Hiroko. 2002. Rural Regions Struggle to Stem Elderly Suicides. *Japan Times*, 8 March.

Nelson, John K. 1996. *A Year in the Life of a Shinto Shrine.* Seattle: University of Washington Press.

Norbeck, Edward. 1953. Age-Grading in Japan. *American Anthropologist* 55:373–383.

Norbeck, Edward. 1954. *Takashima: A Japanese Fishing Community.* Salt Lake City: University of Utah Press.

Ochiai, Emiko. 1997. *The Japanese Family System in Transition: A Sociological Analysis of Family Change in Postwar Japan.* Tokyo: LTCB International Library Foundation.

Ogasawara, Yuko. 1998. *Office Ladies and Salaried Men: Power, Gender, and Work in Japanese Companies.* Berkeley: University of California Press.

Ohnuki-Tierney, Emiko. 1984. *Illness and Culture in Contemporary Japan: An Anthropological View*. New York: Cambridge University Press.

Ooms, Herman. 1967. The Religion of the Household: A Case Study of Ancestor Worship in Japan. *Contemporary Religions in Japan* 8:201–333.

Plath, David W. 1964. "Where the Family of God Is the Family: The Role of the Dead in Japanese Households." *American Anthropologist* 66:300–317.

Plath, David W. 1980. *Long Engagements: Maturity in Modern Japan*. Stanford: Stanford University Press.

Puette, William J. 1983. *The Tale of Genji: A Reader's Guide*. Rutland, VT: Charles E. Tuttle Co.

Rappaport, Roy A. 1999. *Ritual and Religion in the Making of Humanity*. New York: Cambridge University Press.

Raymo, James M. 1998. Later Marriages or Fewer? Changes in the Marital Behavior of Japanese Women. *Journal of Marriage and the Family* 60 (November 1998):1023–1034.

Reader, Ian. 1990. *Religion in Contemporary Japan*. Honolulu: University of Hawaii Press.

Reader, Ian. 1991. Letters to the Gods: The Form and Meaning of Ema. *Japanese Journal of Religious Studies* 18(1):23–50.

Reader, Ian and George J. Tanabe, Jr. 1998. *Practically Religious: Worldly Benefits and the Common Religion of Japan*. Honolulu: University of Hawaii Press.

Rice, Yoshie Noshioka. 2001. The Maternal Role in Japan: Cultural Values and Socioeconomic Conditions. In Hidetada Shimizu and Robert A. Levine (eds.), *Japanese Frames of Mind: Cultural Perspectives on Human Development*. New York: Cambridge University Press. Pp. 85–110.

Rimer, J. Thomas. 1976. *Four Plays by Tanaka Chikao*. Monumenta Nipponica 31(3):275–298.

Roberts, John M., Saburo Morita, and L. Keith Brown. 1986. Personal Categories for Japanese Sacred Places and Gods: Views Elicited from a Conjugal Pair. *American Anthropologist* 88:807–824.

Rorty, Richard. 1979. *Philosophy and the Mirror of Nature.* Princeton: Princeton University Press.

Rorty, Richard. 1989. *Contingency, Irony, and Solidarity.* Cambridge: Cambridge University Press.

Rowe, John W. and Robert L. Kahn. 1998. *Successful Aging.* New York: Dell Publishing.

Saltonstall, Robin. 1993. Healthy Bodies, Social Bodies: Men's and Women's Concepts and Practices of Health in Everyday Life. *Social Science and Medicine* 36(1):7–14.

Sanjek, Roger. Ed. 1990. *Fieldnotes: The Making of Anthropology.* Ithaca: Cornell University Press.

Sargent, Carolyn. 1991. Women's Roles and Women Healers in Contemporary Rural and Urban Benin. In Carol Shepherd McClain (ed.), *Women as Healers: Cross-Cultural Perspectives.* New Brunswick: Rutgers University Press. Pp. 204–218.

Sato, Eiko et al. 1992. *Kanegasaki-chō shi (The History of Kanegasaki).* Kanegasaki: Kanegasaki Town Government.

Schnell, Scott. 1995. Ritual as an Instrument of Political Resistance in Rural Japan. *Journal of Anthropological Research* 51:301–328.

Schnell, Scott. 1999. *The Rousing Drum: Ritual Practice in a Japanese Community.* Honolulu: University of Hawaii Press.

Schrag, Calvin O. 1997. *The Self after Postmodernity.* New Haven: Yale University Press.

Singleton, John. 1993. Gambaru: *A Japanese Cultural Theory of Learning.* In *Japanese Schooling: Patterns of Socialization, Equality, and Political Control.* James J. Shields, ed. Pp. 8–15. University Park: The Pennsylvania State University Press.

Sloan, Richard P. 2001. Spirituality and Medical Practice: A Look at the Evidence. *American Family Physician* 63(1):33.

Sloan, Richard P., E. Bagiella, and T. Powell. 1999. Religion, Spirituality, and Medicine. *Lancet* 353:664–7.

Smith, Robert J. 1974. *Ancestor Worship in Contemporary Japan.* Stanford: Stanford University Press.

Smith, Robert J. 1984. *Japanese Society: Tradition, Self, and the Social Order.* New York: Cambridge University Press.

Smith, Wilfred Cantwell. 1977. *Belief and History.* Charlottesville: University Press of Virginia.

Smyers, Karen. 1997. Inari Pilgrimage: Following One's Own Path on the Mountain. *Japanese Journal of Religious Studies* 24(3–4):427–452.

Smyers, Karen A. 1999. *The Fox and the Jewel: Shared and Private Meanings in Contemporary Japanese Inari Worship.* Honolulu: University of Hawaii Press.

Sōmuchō (Statistics Bureau, Japanese Government). 1998. *Kōreika Shakai Hakusho* [White Paper on the Aging Society]. Tokyo: ōkurashō insatsu kyoku. Sōmuchō tōkei kyoku [Statistics Bureau, Management and Coordination Agency (Japanese Government)].

Sōmuchō (Statistics Bureau, Japanese Government). 2000. *Kōreika Shakai Hakusho* [White Paper on the Aging Society]. Tokyo: ōkurashō insatsu kyoku. Sōmuchō tōkei kyoku [Statistics Bureau, Management and Coordination Agency (Japanese Government)].

Strathern, Andrew. 1989. Melpa Dream Interpretation and the Concept of Hidden Truth. *Ethnology* 28:301–315.

Suzuki, Hikaru. 1998. Japanese Death Rituals in Transit: From Household Ancestors to Beloved Antecedents. *Journal of Contemporary Religion* 13(2):171–188.

Swyngedouw, Jan. 1993. "Religion in Contemporary Japanese Society." Pp. 49–72 In *Religion and Society in Modern Japan*, edited by Mark R. Mullins, Shimazono Susumu, and Paul L. Swanson. Berkeley: Asian Humanities Press.

Tamanoi, Mariko Asano. 1998. *Under the Shadow of Nationalism: Politics and Poetics of Rural Japanese Women*. Honolulu: University of Hawaii Press.

Thomas, L. Eugene and Susan A. Eisenhandler (eds.). 1999. *Religion, Belief, and Spirituality in Late Life*. New York: Springer Publishing Company.

Tillich, Paul. 1951. *Systematic Theology, Volume One*. Chicago: University of Chicago Press.

Totman, Conrad. 1981. *Japan before Perry: A Short History*. Berkeley: University of California Press.

Traphagan, John W. 1998a. Localizing Senility: Illness and Agency among Older Japanese. *Journal of Cross-Cultural Gerontology* 13(1):81–98.

Traphagan, John W. 1998b. Emic Weeds or Etic Wild Flowers? Structuring the Environment in a Japanese Town. In *Toward Sustainable Cities: Readings in the Anthropology of Urban Environments*. K. Aoyagi, P. J. M. Nas, J. W. Traphagan, eds. Pp. 37–52. Leiden: Institute of Cultural and Social Studies, University of Leiden.

Traphagan, John W. 1998c. Contesting the Transition to Old Age in Japan. *Ethnology* 37(4):333–50.

Traphagan, John W. 2000a. *Taming Oblivion: Aging Bodies and the Fear of Senility in Japan*. Albany: State University of New York Press.

Traphagan, John W. 2000b. The Liminal Family: Return Migration and Intergenerational Conflict in Japan. *Journal of Anthropological Research* Vol. 56, pp. 365–385.

Traphagan, John W. 2000c. Reproducing Elder Male Power through Ritual Performance in Japan. *Journal of Cross-Cultural Gerontology* 15(2):81–97.

Traphagan, John W. 2002. Senility as Disintegrated Person in Japan. *Journal of Cross-Cultural Gerontology* 17(3):253–267.

Traphagan, John W. 2003a. Contesting Co-Residence: Women, In-Laws, and Health Care in Rural Japan. In J. W. Traphagan and

J. Knight (eds.) *Demographic Change and the Family in Japan's Aging Society.* Albany: State University of New York Press.

Traphagan, John W. 2003b. Older Women as Caregivers and Ancestral Protection in Rural Japan. *Ethnology* 42(2):127–140.

Traphagan, John W. 2004. Curse of the Successor: Filial Piety vs. Marriage among Rural Japanese. In Charlotte Ikels (ed.) *Filial Piety: Practice and Discourse in Contemporary East Asia.* Stanford: Stanford University Press.

Traphagan, John W. Forthcoming a. Moral Discourse and Old Age Disability in Japan. In B. Ingstad and S. R. Whyte (eds.) *Disability in Local and Global Worlds.*

Traphagan, John W. Forthcoming b. Being a Good Rōjin: Senility, Power, and Self-Actualization in Japan. In preparation for an edited volume on senility and culture, Lawrence Cohen and Annette Leibing, eds.

Traphagan, John W. and L. Keith Brown. 2002. Fast Food and Intergenerational Commensality in Japan: New Styles and Old Patterns. *Ethnology* 41(2):119–134.

Turner, Victor. 1977. *The Ritual Process.* Ithaca: Cornell University Press.

Tylor, Edward B. 1873. *Primitive Culture: Researches into the Development of Mythology, Philosophy, Religion, Language, Art, and Custom.* Vol 1., 2nd ed. London: John Murray.

Van Gennep, Arnold. 1960. *The Rites of Passage.* M. B. Vizedom and G. L. Cafee, transl. Chicago: University of Chicago Press.

Vogel, Ezra F. 1963. *Japan's New Middle Class.* Berkeley: University of California Press.

Weber, Max. 1963. *The Sociology of Religion.* Ephram Rischoff, trans. Boston: Beacon Press.

Wittgenstein, Ludwig. 1969. *On Certainty.* G. E. M. Anscombe and G. H. von Wrigh, eds. New York: Harper & Row.

Wöss, Fleur. 1993. Pokkuri Temples and Aging: Ritual for Approaching Death. In M. R. Mullins, S. Susumu, and P. L. Swanson, eds. *Religion and Society in Modern Japan.* Pp. 191–202. Berkeley, Calif.: Asian Humanities Press.

Yanagita, Kunio. 1970. Ema to Uma. In *Teihon Yanagita Kunio shū* [Definitive Collected Works of Yanagita Kunio], 27:341–43. Tokyo: Chikuma Shobō.

Yiengpruksawan, Mim Hall. 1998. *Hiraizumi: Buddhist Art and Regional Politics in Twelfth-Century Japan.* Cambridge: Harvard University Asia Center.

Yoshida, Mitsuhiro. 1997. *Contesting powers: A Cultural Analysis of Water Distribution, Personhood, Gender and Ritual in a Japanese Hot Spring Town.* Doctoral dissertation. Department of Anthropology, University of Pittsburgh.

Index